# THIS
# IS HOW
# YOUR
# MARRIAGE
# ENDS

*A Hopeful Approach to
Saving Relationships*

# MATTHEW FRAY

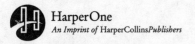
HarperOne
*An Imprint of* HarperCollins*Publishers*

# THIS
# IS HOW
# YOUR
# MARRIAGE
# ENDS

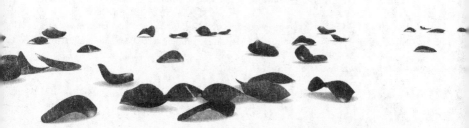

HarperCollins books may be purchased for educational, business, or sales promotional use. For information, please email the Special Markets Department at SPsales@harpercollins.com.

*Illustration by Fedorov Ivan Sergeevich / Shutterstock*

Library of Congress Cataloging-in-Publication Data is available upon request.

ISBN 978-0-06-307226-8

24 25 26 27 28  LBC  7 6 5 4 3

*To my son. Be better than your father. Please work to be what you and your mom deserved from me. Be kind, even when it's hard. Painful things will sometimes happen. For you and those you love. Darkness will occasionally fall because it always does. When that happens, you be the light.*

*To his mother. This is—for better or worse, for richer or poorer—for you. Because it can't not be. I'm so sorry.*

# CONTENTS

INTRODUCTION: The Stories We Tell Ourselves                    1

CHAPTER 1: This Is How Your Marriage Ends                      11

CHAPTER 2: Good People Can Be Bad Spouses                      37

CHAPTER 3: The Invalidation Triple Threat:
The Danger Hiding in the Shadows                               63

CHAPTER 4: Is Your Spouse Hurting You on Purpose?              87

CHAPTER 5: Words Don't Always Mean What
We Think They Mean                                            123

CHAPTER 6: Move the Dots Closer: Key Relationship
Skills to Practice and Master                                 151

CHAPTER 7: Marriage and the Man Card                          183

CHAPTER 8: She Feels Like Your Mom and
Doesn't Want to . . .                                         213

CHAPTER 9: Sex, Lies, and Internet Porn                       237

CHAPTER 10: What Matters vs. What Doesn't                    265

CONCLUSION: The Art of Getting to Tomorrow                   287

ACKNOWLEDGMENTS                                             295

# INTRODUCTION:
## THE STORIES WE TELL OURSELVES

A MAN FALLS INTO A HOLE WITH WALLS TOO HIGH TO CLIMB.

He's hurt and afraid.

*"Please help!"* he cries. *"I'm stuck down here!"*

Just then a doctor walks by and, hearing the cries for help, writes a prescription and drops it into the hole before moving along.

*"Somebody! Anybody! Please help me!"*

Next, a pastor walking by stops, scribbles a prayer onto a piece of paper, pitches it down to the trapped man, and continues on.

*"I need help! I can't get out!"* the man shouts.

Finally, a friend walks by, sees the man trapped in the hole, and immediately jumps in as well.

*"You idiot! Now you're down here too! Why would you do that?!"* the man asks.

His friend replies: "Because I've been down here before. I may know the way out. And because I want you to know you're not alone."

○

I was thirty-four and crying more than an adult man probably should. Because my wife left. And because I missed our little boy who was no longer home every day. And because she was seeing some dickbag who holds the distinction of being the only human I ever wished would die in a fiery explosion.

Even though I'd barely touched my wife in the previous two years, the thought of someone else doing so wrecked me. My young son, not yet in kindergarten, would now be raised by this dickbag, I thought. *I no longer have any agency over who gets to look after my son.* I imagined a future where he would run off the field after Little League games and jump into the arms of his mom and evil stepdad, who would look to everyone else like a beautiful little family. And I'd be some distance away, forcing a polite smile as if everything were okay but secretly wishing I were dead.

But I also had other immediate problems to deal with. After a lifetime of living with parents, college roommates, or my wife, I was for the first time without companionship. That wouldn't do.

Stories abound of guys my age being released back into the wild. Cleaning up in the dating world armed with the confidence and sexual competence that comes with the life and bedroom experience we don't possess in our formative years. *I should try online dating! People don't make fun of you for that anymore!*

I tried online dating on Match and Tinder, despite Tinder's reputation at the time as being an app for cheap hook-ups.

Mostly, women weren't interested. Because the internet allows people to easily filter their dating preferences, it didn't take long to realize that recently divorced, 5'9" single fathers who cry a lot aren't considered the cream of the online dating crop.

But there were a few takers. The widow who liked me but chastised me for being on online dating sites despite being emotionally unavailable so soon after divorce. The hearing specialist who texted 'LOL' after every.single.typed.sentence. The woman who turned out to be the sister of a guy I knew at work, which led both of us to shake hands and say, "Welp. This is a shit idea. Have a nice life and stuff."

Before a date, I'd coach myself: *Don't talk about your divorce. Don't talk about your divorce. Don't talk about your divorce.* I'd talk about my divorce before the appetizers arrived. *Idiot!*

I sucked ass at dating. Not only did I cry too much but my hair was graying, I was the father of a four-year-old, which instantly weeds out a ton of people disinterested in stepmotherhood, and the politely outraged widow was right: I was there to combat loneliness, not to make authentic human connections that might lead to healthy, sustainable relationships.

I'd think about how unfair it felt that my wife seemed so happy in her new life and relationship while I was binge-watching Netflix through tears, miserable and alone.

*I'm going to die a lonely incel and that shit-eater is going to hug my son and French-kiss my wife next to my casket before he flies them to an amazing African safari vacation where my wife will inevitably celebrate my passing with some uncomfortably hot sex act we never tried and say, "Hahahahahahaha! I bet Matt sat around crying all the time and no girls wanted to kiss him! What a small, little loser he was! I'm so glad I'm here with you instead of him!"*

That's seriously what I thought about. They were dark times.

One night, while freaking out and self-medicating with vodka, I called a therapist on a 1–800 number and I'm pretty sure she thought I was a loser.

She asked me questions about my life. I probably offered, "Umm. I'm getting divorced. I'm involuntarily celibate. I'm pretty sure that some guy I don't know is sticking his penis inside of my wife. Things are awesome. Thanks for asking."

She said, *"Since you're a writer, I think it would be good for you to start a journal. Just write down what you feel."*

She probably meant that I should write things in a private journal. Instead, I got a little drunk and put it on the internet.

## FROM DIVORCE BLOGGER TO RELATIONSHIP COACH TO BOOK AUTHOR

I started the blog *Must Be This Tall To Ride* in 2013 as a means of processing my grief and anger following my divorce per the phone-a-therapist's suggestion. She encouraged me to write my feelings. So, that's what I did. It was supposed to be a dark comedy documenting my trials and tribulations as a recently divorced, midlife-crisis-having single father trying to date and start a new life. I thought it would be funny in a dysfunctionally pathetic way.

I treated it almost like a journal. It was easy to write vulnerably and authentically because I felt too miserable to care what anyone thought of me and because there didn't seem to be any danger of anyone reading it.

But then people totally read it and provided feedback. A small but engaged and growing audience formed.

Those people saved my life in several ways. People liked the writing, they said. It helped them feel less alone, they said. My public self-reflections on marriage and divorce felt personal and familiar to them, they said.

*I'm not the only one*, we discovered collectively.

The fact that people were paying attention changed everything. *Am I going to contribute to the empty-calorie click-bait noise? Or am I going to try to do something that matters?*

I had been writing sad and angry tales of how I felt my ex-wife was mistreating me and being unfair to me and how hard my life was and *me me me me me me me.* Sprinkled with a little more me.

And then on July 3, 2013, during my first out-of-town trip without my wife following our separation, I wrote and published a blog post titled *An Open Letter to Shitty Husbands, Vol. 1.* It's not very good. It wasn't important because of its quality. It was important because it represented a critical shift in the way I had been thinking about my failed marriage.

I began to ask, because I needed to know: *What did I do to make her feel like this was her best option?*

I read several books and articles about the conditions that commonly end relationships. They sounded eerily similar to the end of my marriage. I locked in on the behaviors commonly linked to romantic partners feeling emotionally neglected and abandoned. The kind of behaviors that result in the breakdown of safety and trust in relationships. I spent time self-reflecting, for the first time ever, challenging my own beliefs and assumptions. For the first time ever, I asked myself difficult questions about how much of this horror show was actually because of me.

The answers made me squirm. Call it uncomfortable truth versus comfortable lies.

My wife and I were much like many other husbands and wives, it turns out. Maybe even most. We weren't weird. We weren't freaks. We weren't a statistical anomaly. We were the norm. And that terrified me because I finally knew just how bad divorce can be. It can turn you into a person you don't even recognize anymore. And if my wife and I were the norm? That meant that everyone was in danger.

*How can we expect marriages to last when it appears as if romantic partners aren't even aware of these conditions and behaviors that will eventually end their relationships?*

So, I kept writing my first-person stories about marriage. About how I'd inadvertently damaged my wife. I'd tell a story, and people would say, *"That's exactly like my marriage! I wish my shitty husband would figure this out like you did!"*

People said they could see themselves in my stories. Their partners said that my realizations gave them hope that maybe their spouses could develop the ability to think and speak in this new way.

*"If you can do this, then maybe my husband can do it too. Thank you."*

And then it happened: A married couple wrote to tell me that my stories had helped them recognize and define what was happening in their marriage, and that it had inspired change, ultimately saving their marriage and family.

*Whoa.*

People were using my public self-reflections to look inward and have uncomfortable conversations with themselves and their relationship partners.

Then some of these people were leveraging these shared ideas to grow and change in tangible ways, positively affecting their lives and their loved ones.

So, there I was. Divorced. Single. A total relationship failure by any measure. Yet, people were crediting me with saving their marriages. People were saying that my way of explaining human relationships helped them understand theirs in ways they previously had not.

I had set out to write entertaining stories about a dysfunctional, divorced, single father trying to navigate online dating for the five people who might be interested. I accidentally ended up a self-help writer.

○

Speaker, podcaster, and social media influencer Mark Groves encouraged me to start coaching people.

That sounded like a bad idea. *Who the hell am I to act as if I'm some expert and ask people to pay me for my amateur, divorced-guy guidance?* So, I didn't act on it even though Mark is smart, successful, and was generously providing mentorship.

A year later, Mark and I were back on the phone and he was patiently repeating his suggestion for me to coach people. He heard my resistance, then pointed out the obvious. I wasn't advertising. I wasn't encouraging people to choose me over more traditional forms of relationship therapy or couples counseling. I was simply making myself available to people who were already on my website, reading my articles, and connecting with the stories.

So—even though I was terrified—I started coaching people who asked me to work with them. We talk on the phone or via online videoconferencing. It turns out that, when you do things over and over again, they get less scary.

After a year of working one-on-one with coaching clients, I was asked by *New York Times* writer Jancee Dunn (author of *How Not to Hate Your Husband After Kids* and many other books) to participate in a feature article about my work. It turns out that I'm on a short list of male non-mental-health professionals who talk and write about relationships in the way that I do.

The *New York Times* story ran in May 2020 in the early stages of the COVID-19 pandemic—when many married and dating couples were locked down at home together, exacerbating strained relationships globally.

Exposure from the *Times* article led to offers to create unscripted television shows, and several media interview requests from around the world—from Ryan Seacrest's radio show in Los Angeles, California, to *Die Zeit* in Hamburg, Germany.

And now I have been given the opportunity to write this book. I hope you like some of it.

**My overarching premise is that good people who want to be married accidentally hurt one another and betray each other's trust without either partner being aware of it as it is happening until their marriage slowly becomes toxic and/or ends.**

Just as health professionals in the 1950s and '60s were compelled to sound the alarm regarding the dangers of tobacco smoking to a then-unaware public, this book's purpose is to raise awareness of routine, everyday behaviors happening in marriage (or any long-term romantic relationship) that will lead to relationship sickness and death if gone unchecked.

Because how can these things ever be dealt with or fixed if people don't realize they're a problem?

The conditions that end marriages and keep the divorce rate sky-high are the results of unremarkable, everyday behaviors. Behaviors most people perceive to be so ordinary and inconsequential that they don't know to be afraid of them, how to avoid them, how to discuss them effectively, or how to repair the damage caused by them (often because at least one of us spends most of our energy denying anything's wrong in the first place).

We often fail to identify the real root causes of our broken relationships, which then dooms us to repeat the same behaviors in future relationships. (Which explains the nearly 70 percent divorce rate in second marriages.)

A resource for couples who are dating before marriage or are currently married or for people like me who divorced and want to know why, this book's aim is to help you identify relationship-killing behavior patterns and communication habits in your life and point you toward new ideas, skills, and resources to help your relationships thrive.

There are no one-size-fits-all answers for any of this. Common patterns emerge in relationships. Some good. Some not. And they happen in every place on earth. These toxic relationship patterns transcend language, skin color, geography, religion, age, and sexual orientation.

Everywhere on earth people voluntarily enter loving, monogamous relationships. The vast majority won't make it no matter how much they want to.

We can do better.

I hope this book can help readers develop some of the emotional-intelligence skills and awareness required to have healthy and successful long-term relationships.

I'm not going to attempt this with any holier-than-thou preachiness. I won't judge you nor will I act as if I think I'm smart and awesome and that you're some moron who needs my help.

I got most of it wrong. Relationship stuff. Marriage. I was terrible but had no idea I was terrible as life was happening.

This is the story of how I came to understand the many ways that I emotionally neglected and abandoned my wife in our marriage all while convincing myself she was the one most responsible for our relationship problems. This is the story of how I hurt my wife with a smile on my face, honestly believing that I was a good guy being treated unfairly every time she acted sad or wounded.

And I wish this were my story and no one else's. But this is the story of marriage everywhere. Millions of people. Maybe billions.

But it doesn't have to be.

# 1

# THIS IS HOW YOUR MARRIAGE ENDS

This is the way your marriage ends, this is the way your marriage ends, this is the way your marriage ends.
Not with a bang but a whimper.

*APOLOGIES TO T. S. ELIOT

## THE FISH SANDWICH INCIDENT

"Everything is shut down right now because of the pandemic," he said. "I was starving and really busy with work. So, I got a fish sandwich, and now my wife is going to freak out about it."

He wasn't *starving*-starving. Just hungrier than normal and prone to the sort of hyperbole many of us think and speak with. An unexpected "work emergency" in real estate had forced Grayson to miss both breakfast and lunch. He was getting that empty-stomach sick feeling and wanted food.

It was the spring of 2020 and his Connecticut town was largely shut down, including most restaurants, due to the COVID-19 pandemic. Finding a quick meal in those conditions might have been simple for most of us, but because Grayson and his wife adhered to a strict vegan diet—which excludes any animal-derived products, including all meat, eggs, and dairy—Grayson's food-acquisition efforts were more complicated.

Oh! And one other thing: Vegan diets also exclude fish.

Grayson was one of my relationship coaching clients. There was conflict at home. His wife was perpetually angry with him, he said, and he wanted help figuring out why and what he could do about it.

I called him at our scheduled appointment time on what happened to be the same afternoon as The Fish Sandwich Incident.

"Dude. You gotta help me out," he said. "I don't know what to say to my wife. She's going to be all pissed off and up my ass."

I laughed even though I take marital conflict seriously.

He said his wife had just been texting him, asking what he had eaten for lunch. The truth would cause another fight. This is what always happens, he said. His wife is always overreacting, he said. It's as if he can never predict the next thing that will upset her.

Everything Grayson was experiencing made sense to me because his story sounded a lot like the stories I might have told a decade earlier when I was still married. How it seemed as if my wife was quick to complain or criticize me about things that I had the good decency to peacefully let go of whenever the roles were reversed.

*I'm so nice,* I'd think. *Why doesn't she notice how nice I am? If she were as nice to me as I am to her, we'd probably never fight at all!*

I can't know what people truly thought about me, but for the better part of thirty years, I perceived myself to be both likable and well-liked. Even if I were delusional, it still felt good. Being the kind of person people like made more sense to me and seemed more appealing to me than being someone people didn't like.

Maybe that's why I'd feel so angry when my wife would act as if she didn't like me.

*No good deed is ever enough. No sacrifice I make proves my commitment. No amount of love nor any kindness I feel or display is ever acknowledged.*

I never felt more unappreciated or more unfairly treated than the times my wife would communicate some new way in which I had disappointed her. It felt as if the girl I loved and married had arbitrarily adjusted her standards for what was okay and not okay.

I hadn't changed. She had. And it didn't seem fair that she had "roped me into marriage" under the pretense that we were great for one another and loved each other as we were, but years later, I was no longer good enough.

*This is bullshit*, I'd think.

And Grayson was now living through a similar scenario, and it felt like bullshit to him too.

"What was I supposed to do?" he said.

Grayson was genuinely busy with work the day of The Fish Sandwich Incident—he had to eat quickly so he could keep his appointment. That was real and immediate. There was a global pandemic happening that had changed everyday life, including the shutdown of local restaurants. And under those circumstances, it makes sense that finding a vegan meal might be difficult. He did the best that he could. Fish sandwiches do tend to be healthier options than bacon double cheeseburgers.

And much like him, I simply cannot imagine being upset with someone for eating a fish sandwich. Absent context, I consider it unhealthy to get angry over the type of sandwich someone eats.

"So, what do I do, man? This is the kind of shit she's always getting mad about and it's so frustrating," he said. "Why can't she understand the situation I was in and give me the benefit of the doubt?"

After assuring Grayson that I could relate to his frustration, I asked whether he and his wife had an agreement with one another to be vegan. I wanted to know whether—from his wife's perspective—promises had been made regarding their eating habits.

"Definitely," he said. "I've told her that I would do this with her and that I would be disciplined with my diet. But man, it was just fish, and like I said before, none of the restaurants were open."

"I get all of this," I told him. "But we need to be fair to your wife. Because it's going to be really easy to go meet your buddies for a round of golf this weekend and tell them all about how your naggy wife freaked out over a fish sandwich a few days ago."

Surely, one or all of them would have nodded their heads knowingly because their romantic partners do insane, inexplicable things just like that.

"Sorry, man," one might say. "My old lady is the exact same way. Always getting pissed off over little things that don't even matter."

But that nagging-wife story is complete nonsense.

Characterizing my client's wife as losing her mind over him eating a fish sandwich is EXACTLY the kind of intellectually lazy story I told years ago. I felt as if my wife used to go off the deep end over petty stuff just like fish sandwiches. And because she did that, and I didn't lose it over "silly things," I perceived myself to be the mature one. I was fair-minded. Levelheaded. Smart. And she was someone who didn't know how to maintain a healthy perspective. She was someone who couldn't even tell the difference between a stupid fish sandwich and things that actually mattered.

"Your wife believes you to be someone who avoids eating certain foods because it's a promise that you both made to one another?" I asked. "It's a code that you two live by? Something you are doing together as a team, because you perceive it to be healthy living and the sort of behavior you want to model for your kids?"

Yes, he said.

"So, let's please be careful about how we think and speak about this," I said. "Your wife isn't acting like some crazy lunatic who is freaking out because you ate a fish sandwich. Your wife is acting like someone who has just been hurt. Grayson, your wife is hurt because she just experienced betrayal. She doesn't give a shit about the fish sandwich, and it's disingenuous and dishonest to run around characterizing her that way."

What Grayson's wife actually gave a shit about was being married to someone who keeps promises. If she is married to someone she perceives to be unwilling or unable to keep their promises, then there can't be trust in the relationship. A relationship absent trust doesn't feel safe because relationships without trust are unsustainable. People require safety. We need safety to function, else we focus time and effort on trying to eliminate the threat or flee to safety.

Maybe that's evacuating a building during a fire alarm. Maybe that's running away from hungry lions. Maybe that's fleeing a city about to be hit by a hurricane.

Or maybe that's divorcing someone unwilling or unable to fulfill the requirements of maintaining trust in a marriage.

Grayson's wife wasn't upset because her husband ate fish. Grayson's wife was upset because her husband made a decision that betrayed her trust, and adding insult to injury, he followed it up by leveraging her anger as an example of what an unfair, nagging asshole she can be "when she doesn't get her way."

Grayson's story reminded me of conversations my wife and I used to have about things like me leaving a dish by the sink or about me tossing an item of clothing on a piece of furniture in our bedroom.

It felt unfair to Grayson to be chastised for something as seemingly benign as eating a fish sandwich under extraordinary circumstances. And it felt deeply painful to his wife to discover that her husband had broken a promise.

Sometimes, in human relationships, conversations about fish sandwiches are actually conversations about painful betrayals. Our failure to recognize it dooms us to repeating the same arguments and finding ourselves in maddeningly circular conversations over and over again until something breaks painfully enough for us to notice.

Something is wrong, they say. *No, it's not.*

Something hurts, they say. *No, it doesn't.*

I can't live like this, they say. *It's so unfair that I'm always made out to be the bad guy and that nothing I do is ever good enough.*

These are two decent, kind, intelligent, well-meaning people who love one another, and—philosophically—want their marriage to succeed. Yet, no matter how hard they try to explain themselves to one another, nothing seems to get better. The hurt keeps growing slowly in intensity as frustration mounts and resentment grows.

Home lives and partnerships that once felt safe and comfortable slowly morph into a life that does not.

Relationships with people whom we trusted when they promised to love us forever no longer feel trustworthy.

We will explore these ideas further in later chapters, but it is the erosion and eventual loss of safety and trust that create the conditions for the death of a marriage.

John Lennon and Sir Paul McCartney famously wrote and sang

"All You Need Is Love" as members of The Beatles in 1967. Maybe they even believed it at the time.

I'm here to argue that love—romantic love—is, at best, maybe the No. 4 most important ingredient for a marriage or long-term committed relationship capable of going the distance.

## DIVORCE: THE GREAT SOCIAL CRISIS OF OUR TIME

There is no greater threat to people's health and wellness than toxic relationships and divorce. Living in a broken marriage or going through divorce is one of the most disruptive and painful experiences a person will encounter in their lifetime. Worse still, it's LIKELY to happen.

1. Statistically, 95 percent of Americans ages eighteen and older fall into one of three categories—married, formerly married, or intending to marry in the future.

2. About 70 percent of people who marry will suffer from a dysfunctional relationship and/or from its eventual end. (This 70 percent figure accounts for the people who end up divorced as well as the people who remain married but are unhappy within their marriages.)

3. Divorce and marital separation rank Nos. 2 and 3, respectively, as being the most stressful life events a person can experience, according to psychologists studying the impact of stress on physical health. My less-scientific way of measuring divorce in terms of the amount of crying and anxiety-induced vomiting I experienced corroborates the researchers' findings.

4. The conditions that cause marriages or long-term romantic relationships to deteriorate from positive and healthy to negative and unhealthy are very subtle. I'll go as far as to call them invisible.

5. Conclusion: Virtually everyone is affected by the negative consequences of shitty marriages and divorce. The information and life skills required for people to participate effectively in healthy, sustainable romantic relationships appear to be missing from the majority of people's skill sets and vocabularies. It's nobody's fault. It's our responsibility, of course. But not our fault. Neither our parents nor our grandparents taught us these things or even talked about them in a way that prepared us for the rigors of adult relationships. But don't blame them, please. No one taught them either.

Common themes emerge from people's divorce stories.

The relationship becomes strained but not quickly nor obviously. The strain sneaks in slowly. Quietly. Insidiously. If we recognized what was happening as it was happening, most of us would course-correct, since most of us legitimately love our spouses and want our marriages to succeed.

We're not intentionally sabotaging our most important relationships. We're accidentally doing it. Most of us don't even know it's happening as it's happening. They're not bombs and gunshots—these moments that contribute to the gradual breakdown of our relationships. They're pinpricks. They're paper cuts.

These tiny wounds don't kill us instantly nor trigger any sense of danger. And THAT is the danger. When we don't recognize something as threatening, then we're not on guard. We don't make preparations or adjustments to protect ourselves and others from potentially horrible outcomes.

These tiny wounds start to bleed, and the bleed-out is so gradual that many of us don't recognize the threat until it's too late to stop it.

Divorce was very difficult for me and I believe it is very difficult for most of us. But it's not something we spend a lot of time discussing. Maybe it's because we're ashamed or maybe it's because divorce conversations are awkward and uncomfortable to be on either side of.

My wife and I mostly pretended that everything was okay when other people were around. I didn't want people to know that my marriage was falling apart. I don't know how much of that was politeness and how much of it was fear. It felt a lot like the times I have been in financial trouble but didn't want anyone knowing about it. Whether as a couple or as an individual, when I was invited to join friends on a vacation trip, or more simply to a nice restaurant for a weekend night out, more often than not, I didn't have the money to say yes. (Or I would say yes knowing there would be a shortage for paying bills and life expenses later.)

Sometimes we don't tell the truth—not to be gross and deceptive in a con-artisty way—but maybe to avoid advertising the shame we're trying to hide or to politely spare the people we love from our baggage.

People often don't feel invited to share the scariest, most stressful parts of their lives. And while we're all walking around wearing our politeness masks or trying to hide things we're ashamed of, millions of people live under the mistaken belief that we're the only ones dealing with the stress and fear and sadness and anger we feel.

O

When we remove the visceral experience of living through a crumbling relationship on the brink of ending and think about the state of marriage and long-term romantic relationships on a macro level, our detachment naturally becomes even more pronounced.

Breakups are common. Divorce is common.

Thousands happen every day. Common things seem normal. Regular. Not weird. And things we think of as common typically do not scare us. Then, because we're not afraid of anything bad happening, we often fail to protect or prepare ourselves. When we see people taking protective action before marriage, it's often in the form of a legal prenuptial (or antenuptial) agreement mostly designed to protect one relationship partner from being betrayed or taken advantage of financially by the person they're marrying if the marriage is later dissolved.

Outside of prenups and a little bit of pre-marriage counseling common in certain religions, most people enter marriage having spent little to no time preparing themselves in any meaningful way. When I imagined being married, I pictured it looking and feeling like a continuation of the few years we had already spent together. When it comes to long-term relationships other than marriage, even less attention is given to preparation.

*Marriage is just like being Forever Boyfriend and Forever Girlfriend! This is gonna be great!*

We enter marriage totally unaware that unpleasant preexisting conditions in our dating relationships that we calculate to be tolerable or something that might dissipate in time will often metastasize in marriage and eventually kill whatever we used to be.

We do not know what will end our relationships and typically lack the tools and skills we need to mitigate these problems even if we did know.

We are set up to fail in our most critical, foundational human relationships. We don't actually know that we're not getting it right, else we'd make much different choices. But it never occurs to us that we should.

*Everything's fine. This will all blow over soon.*

## LOSING A SPOUSE: THE MOST STRESSFUL LIFE EVENT PEOPLE EXPERIENCE

In 1967, psychiatrists Thomas Holmes and Richard Rahe were studying the health impact of various life events on people by examining the stressful "weight" of each event on the lives of their patients.

The result of Holmes and Rahe's work was the Social Readjustment Rating Scale, also called the Holmes-Rahe Stress Inventory or the Holmes and Rahe Stress Scale.

As mentioned previously, their research concluded that divorce is the No. 2 most-stressful life event a person can experience, ahead of things like going to prison, the death of a parent or child, and losing a body part in a horrific accident. **Note:** *Holmes and Rahe were measuring stress specifically, not the intensity of the emotional or psychological trauma. Event A might HURT more than Event B, but Event B can still produce more physical stress on our minds and bodies.*

Only the death of a spouse ranks higher as a life stressor. It's not a coincidence that losing a spouse by any means sits atop the stress meter.

A marital separation or divorce changes your life overnight.

There are legal and financial concerns. Maybe there are children and pets. Family gatherings can never be the same. Social happenings aren't what they used to be.

## The Holmes-Rahe Life Stress Inventory
### THE SOCIAL READJUSTMENT RATING SCALE

INSTRUCTIONS: Mark down the point value of each of these life events that has happened to you during the previous year. Total these associated points. Over 150 points indicates an elevated risk of developing a stress-related illness. Over 300 suggests a high risk, so please take care of yourself.

| LIFE EVENT | MEAN VALUE |
|---|---|
| 1. Death of spouse | 100 |
| 2. Divorce | 73 |
| 3. Marital separation from mate | 65 |
| 4. Detention in jail or other institution | 63 |
| 5. Death of a close family member | 63 |
| 6. Major personal injury or illness | 53 |
| 7. Marriage | 50 |
| 8. Being fired at work | 47 |
| 9. Marital reconciliation with mate | 45 |
| 10. Retirement from work | 45 |
| 11. Major change in the health or behavior of a family member | 44 |
| 12. Pregnancy | 40 |
| 13. Revision of personal habits (dress manners, associations, quitting smoking) | 24 |
| 14. Changes in residence | 20 |
| 15. Major change in sleeping habits (a lot more or less than usual) | 16 |

TOTAL _____

Part of your identity gets stripped away and you don't even get to be you anymore. Everything hurts. You cry. You feel ashamed. Afraid. Insecure. Guilty. And then you cry some more.

○

I'm admittedly confused about why we're not having this conversation more loudly and in greater numbers.

How can it be that we have entire education systems dedicated to teaching children and young adults important subject matter and skill building but we don't address interpersonal romantic relationships that affect virtually everyone?

Statistically speaking, 95 out of 100 people will get married, or are planning to. Of the remaining 5 percent, I think it's safe to assume that many will, at various times in adulthood, be in long-term romantic relationships, the dynamics of which will often mirror marriage.

Let's recap the most statistically common real-world scenario between a man and a woman:

A couple meets. Ages range from teens to people in their forties, but most are in their twenties when they meet the person they will marry.

Usually, these young people feeling totally in love and considering a life together are not maladjusted, criminally inclined psychopaths, pathological liars, violent, sick, stupid, or evil. Most of the time, they're two generally kind, decent people who fall in love and volunteer to marry one another (*they do it on purpose because they WANT to*). Both people conceptually understand the terms of marriage. That it is a life-long commitment, and that if either of them messes it up, life could get pretty terrible for everyone involved. Both are also aware that nearly half of all marriages end in divorce, but no one believes they will be among the divorced half.

In other words, while we are emotionally ill-prepared for what's coming, pretty much everyone is intellectually aware of what they're agreeing to when they voluntarily enter marriage.

In the United States, 99 out of 100 accepted marriage proposals begin with the future groom popping the question. He's just a young man with a dream. He's statistically likely to be twenty-nine and to have spent more than $6,000 on the engagement ring.

The happy, optimistic couple begin to plan the wedding. They will typically invite most of the people they know to their wedding ceremony and reception—a one-day party on which the couples or their parents will shell out on average—wait for it—$30,000.

The sum of money and guest-invitation list might seem superficial in the context of two people exchanging wedding vows, but it's important to consider what it means when people are willing to spend that kind of money and make a public declaration of that magnitude to one another in front of everyone they know.

It demonstrates sufficient evidence that these two people are serious about their intentions. That in the months leading up to their wedding, and on the day itself, they considered their many options and settled on promising to faithfully love one another for the rest of their lives. They say so in front of an audience—often hundreds of their closest friends and family members, and in addition to that, typically enter a legal marriage contract filed at a nearby courthouse.

These two don't believe they're going to get divorced someday even though it's a well-known fact that marriages end that way about half the time.

In the United States alone, there are about 6,200 marriages per day. The inverse is that there are about 3,000 divorces per day. Think about that for a moment.

More than 6,000 people (a marriage usually involves two partici-pants) plus their children, extended families, friends, and co-workers are dealing with a new divorce every day. Just in the United States. I'd work out the math to calculate all of the shitty marriages and miserable people in other parts of the world as well, but I don't want us to start drinking this early in the book.

Yet, the human spirit is a tough thing to squash. We are resilient and demonstrate a biological or cultural predisposition toward advance-ment and improvement. So, even though divorce is life-shaking and soul-crushing, some dig deep in their bellies down where our guts and courage reside and decide to try again.

*"I'm in love again! Oh, happy day! I've learned so much from my stupid mistakes of the past! I'm going to get married again, and it's going to be everything I always knew marriage could be! I've finally found my soul mate!"*

Perhaps there is less pomp and circumstance the second time around. Maybe people don't usually spend $30,000 and invite a ton of people to their second weddings. I don't pretend to know.

I just know one thing: After all of the life experience and wisdom gained from the previous marriage, and after all of the pain, sadness, and anger felt from the divorce, people in second marriages end them even more often than the inexperienced first-timers who didn't know what they were getting themselves into.

Second marriages in the US fail 67 percent of the time.

○

That's insane, right? That people can go through all of that and then actually do a shittier job of being married the second time? Those ques-tions are rhetorical. OF COURSE, it's insane.

These aren't people with guns to their heads, or even people whose cultural norm is to be subjected to arranged marriages. These are people who, fully understanding concepts like forever and monogamy, are VOLUNTARILY entering marriage with a partner of their choosing.

This is something they want to do and they possess a decent sense of what's at stake, and then it doesn't work half the time. The reward for those who bravely try a second time? About 2:1 odds that they'll be having divorce papers notarized sometime in the not-too-distant future.

## HOW I LEARNED ABOUT DIVORCE

I was a four-year-old only child when I learned what divorce was.

**Disclaimer:** My parents divorced in 1983. I was a little kid who once cried during a tornado drill at my preschool because I thought *The Wizard of Oz* twister was about to swoop in and send us up to the sky. I also did inexplicable things like jam a wad of Scotch tape up one of my nostrils so far during arts and crafts that the teachers couldn't remove it and had to call my mom to leave work and pick me up. We're relying on THAT level of dipshittedness to recall the following events. So maybe take some of the details with a grain of salt. I'm probably getting a bunch of stuff wrong. Here's the part I'm not getting wrong—until my own divorce thirty years later, no life event affected or shaped me as profoundly as this one.

O

Mom and Dad dropped me off at a family friend's home on the day an Iowa divorce court judge would make a custody ruling. They were an older couple who had cool stuff like museum-quality antique miniature wooden ships with functioning masts and sails, a rare Excalibur collector car in the garage, and a little schnauzer or Scottish terrier named Colonel Klink. Presumably after the *Hogan's Heroes* TV show character. I never asked.

We'll be back to get you afterward, my parents said.

*After what?*

We're going to see a judge, they said.

*Why?*

Because Mommy and Daddy aren't going to live together anymore after today, and the judge is going to decide whether you will live here with Dad, or in Ohio with Mom, they said.

*Why?*

I didn't understand what a custody battle was and I doubt anyone tried to explain it. I didn't understand the real-world implications of living hundreds of miles away from one of my parents. I didn't understand the gravity of the judge's decision that day, though there was no choice a court official could make to fix what was broken, or right what was wrong.

After their courtroom visit, my parents returned. Both were sad and crying. I don't think I remember seeing that before.

*Why?*

Dad knelt down to my eye level. The judge decided it would be best for you to live with your mom in Ohio, he said. We'll get to be together during summers and holidays, he said. I will always be your dad and I will always love you, he said. Everything is going to be okay, he said.

Mom knelt down to my eye level. We're moving far away to Ohio to live with your grandparents, she said. I'm so sorry, she said. Your dad will always be your dad and he will always love you, she said. I will never keep you from seeing your dad, she said. We both love you so much, she said. Everything is going to be okay, she said.

*Okay. Can I go play with my toys now?*

I was four. I have a hard-enough time digesting this kind of news today. I needed He-Man and Chewbacca to save the day. I needed my Garfield and E.T. stuffed animals to hug tight.

*Everything is going to be okay.*

I don't remember how much time passed between learning about the judge's decision and my first goodbye to one of my parents. It's often not the details we remember in life's most impactful moments. It's the feeling that sticks.

Maybe you know this one. If you're anything like me, your throat tightens. Almost like there's something stuck inside. It hurts a little. And then a lot. Less of a sting and more of a swelling. You can breathe, but not as easily as you normally do. And you can hide all of that, but you can't hide the tears. The tears give you away every time.

It was time to be strong. Like my plastic hero action figures and their animated counterparts saving the day on my Saturday morning cartoons. If I cried, then it would hurt the parent I was saying bye to even more. And if I cried, it would hurt the parent who was driving me far away from the other.

If I cried, I was hurting Mom and Dad no matter what.

Years later, I'd develop the ability to hold it down—down in my throat and stomach where no one can see. But on that day—still only four and without practice—I hadn't mastered pretending yet.

I waved to Dad for as long as I could still see him. He got smaller in the rear window as we drove toward a new home and new life far away.

Maybe I broke a little on the inside after that first goodbye to my father, or maybe it was a time or two later. These were my first encounters with invisible pain.

O

This unusual living arrangement defined my childhood. Growing up with hundreds of miles between me and one of my parents at any given time. Hardly any of the other kids I knew had divorced parents. The one or two who did lived a short drive away from their other parent so everyone saw each other often.

*Divorce is hard,* I thought many times through the years. *I don't know what I'm going to do with my life, but the one thing I'm certain of is that I'm NEVER going to get divorced.*

Because I knew what was at stake. There's nothing as uncomfortable as that lump in your throat. And I'm no quitter.

You know how people would ask you what you wanted to be when you grew up? I never had a definitive answer other than "I know what I don't want to be—a failure. The one thing I am sure of is that I never want to get divorced."

Oops.

## IS DIVORCE REALLY THAT BAD?

You might be thinking: *"C'mon, Matt. The Great Social Crisis of Our Time? Laying it on a little thick, aren't ya? Sure, divorce is bad, but many things happening in the world are much worse!"*

I'm not here to judge your priorities. All kinds of unfortunate things happen to people who deserve better. And with divorce, an argument can be made that it's sometimes actually a good thing (people should have resources for escaping abusive relationships and fundamentally unhealthy marriages), whereas other undesirable societal conditions including poverty, racism, sexism, and various forms of intolerance and bigotry always make things worse.

I'm not trying to rank all the stuff that sucks and, in the process, thoughtlessly trivialize the important fights good people are out there fighting. I am, however, saying divorce is worse than its reputation.

When people get divorced, most of us are like "Of course, they did. Who didn't see that coming? What a shame. So, what are we having for dinner?" before returning to our regularly scheduled program of watching TV and checking our social media feeds.

○

Is divorce or a long-term breakup really THAT bad? Maybe not for everyone. But my divorce was for me. Maybe I was hypersensitive because of my parents' divorce. Maybe I was worried about what my family and friends would think of me for failing at the most important job I had. Maybe I was afraid of being alone. Maybe I just really missed my wife and son.

Yes, for me, it was THAT bad.

In the earliest months after separating, I was still under the delusion that I was the victim. That divorce was something my wife was doing to me. That it was something she was choosing selfishly and unfairly.

Divorce broke me on the inside. Sometimes I'd catch myself staring at my reflection in the mirror after shaving or brushing my teeth. It was every bit as weird as you're imagining. *Who the hell are you?*

Divorce tainted and poisoned most of my adult memories. As if I'd wasted a bunch of my life. As if none of it had mattered. Divorce triggered the greatest sense of pain and loss that I had ever known—something that I had to carry around and hide while trying in vain to function at work, or with friends, or at family gatherings where nothing would or could ever be the same.

Divorce doesn't just rob you of your past. It robs you of your future. Your hopes and dreams? Your plans you were waking up every day and working toward? *Poof.* Whatever I had imagined tomorrow, and five years, and twenty-five years from now to look and feel like could never be.

It was an extremely uncomfortable and disruptive life reset that I wasn't ready for.

Divorce is not the end of the world, but mentally and emotionally it can feel like it as it's happening. Our brains and bodies are perfectly capable of delivering end-of-the-world feelings regardless of how reliably the sun continues to rise and set each day.

And I blamed my wife. For quitting on me. For taking my son away from me just like my dad had been taken from me when I was a child. *She did this to me.*

Our little boy turned five in the initial months following my divorce—the exact age I was when my parents split. It felt poetic to me in an uncomfortable Edgar Allan Poe sort-of way. When I'd drop him off at his mom's house or she would pick him up from mine, I'd get that same swollen, lump-in-my-throat feeling from childhood. The one I'd experience after moving my luggage from one parent's car to the other and then driving away, fighting tears, knowing it would be months before I would see Mom or Dad again.

I was so fucking angry to be feeling those same emotions again thirty years later as a father and abandoned husband. *She did this to me.*

I kind of wanted to die. Not in a suicidal way, exactly. I was feeling a constant and debilitating pain in my head and chest that was sufficiently horrible enough for me to not be afraid of death for the first time ever.

You're fearless because it seems as if nothing can hurt you any worse than you already feel. (An impermanent condition, it turns out. I'm totally paranoid and afraid of dying again. Yay, healing!)

But that first year or so? Mentally and emotionally, I was a little bit like Heath Ledger's portrayal of the Joker in *The Dark Knight* in the scene in which Batman is speeding toward him on the Batpod (the weird, fat-tired motorcycle) and the Joker is walking straight toward him and asking for it.

I remember driving and seeing massive semi-trucks speeding toward me on the highway and sometimes thinking things like *Maybe the driver will fall asleep and cross over the center into oncoming traffic and just take me out.*

*"Come on. I want you to do it. I want you to do it. Hit me. Hit me!"* the Joker yells maniacally at Batman. It was kind of like that, although I never wore murdery face paint nor wielded any automatic weapons.

For the first time in my life, I was experiencing a level of pain that gave me a perspective on why people sometimes end their lives. I was finally feeling enough darkness for that idea to make sense in a way it previously had not. *If I felt like this every day, with no hope that the hurt would ever stop, maybe I wouldn't want to be alive anymore either.*

This was my first post-divorce breakthrough. It was the first time I can specifically remember noticing my own thoughts, feelings, and beliefs about something that "other people" struggle with (emotional pain and thoughts of self-harm or suicide) and then intentionally adjusting my beliefs because of it.

It didn't take long for me to connect the dots as to how these intensely painful feelings I was having might be similar to what my wife had been experiencing and trying to communicate to me while she was fighting for our marriage.

*Holy shit. Feelings can HURT, I thought. And if feelings can hurt this much, and this is how my wife was feeling, and every time she tried to help me understand her pain I responded as if she was dumb, weak, or crazy, all while refusing to adjust any of my behaviors—doesn't it make sense that she wanted to end our marriage? If I were in her position and were experiencing that same level of pain while not receiving any support or concern from her regarding my suffering, wouldn't I have made the same choice that she did?*

I wasn't well-versed on the subject of empathy—which is among the most important life skills needed to succeed in relationships—but so began my journey.

## BROKEN RELATIONSHIPS ARE MOSTLY THE RESULT OF THINGS WE DON'T KNOW

It's not a particularly mind-blowing or sexy thesis. But we don't need to look around very hard to find millions of emotionally distraught and clinically depressed divorcées, and their many innocent children victimized by the broken-home fallout, who would give almost anything to have their families reunited.

We don't need to look very hard to find people who have had quality educations and who showcase masterful skills in their chosen professions but are suffering from their home lives falling apart.

We don't need to look very hard to find people who seem as if they check every box on their My Life Is Awesome checklist but who would trade all of it just to get rid of the pain they feel from the aftermath of a separation from their partner and family.

Even though my parents divorced when I was little, I spent most of my life believing that what ended marriages were behaviors I classify as

Major Marriage Crimes. If murder, rape, and armed robbery are major crimes in the criminal justice system, I viewed sexual affairs, physical spousal abuse, and gambling away the family savings as Major Marriage Crimes.

Because I wasn't committing Major Marriage Crimes, when my wife and I were on opposite sides of an issue, I would suggest that we should agree to disagree. I believed she was wrong—either that she was fundamentally incorrect in her understanding of the situation or that she was treating me unfairly. It always seemed as if the punishment didn't fit the crime—as if she were charging me with premeditated murder when my infraction was something closer to driving a little bit over the speed limit with a burned-out taillight that I didn't even know was burned out.

I wasn't obligated to "agree with her" just because she wanted me to, I'd say.

I felt and said many things like that throughout our twelve-year relationship. Our marriage died a thousand deaths before it was officially buried.

Relationship problems are not usually occurring because of bad people doing bad things to the people they love. Relationship problems crop up among perfectly decent and well-intentioned people who are simply living our lives and failing to recognize that others are experiencing pain while we're busy feeling comfortable and not paying attention.

The circumstances and behaviors that destroy romantic love, erode trust, poison our emotional health, and unknowingly trigger the Countdown to Divorce time bombs in our marriages are often disguised as harmless, innocent, everyday behaviors.

Usually, love doesn't die in a loud, dramatic way.

It's not bright or flashy. The problems hide in the shadows. The pain sneaks in during the quiet moments of isolated disconnection when we are alone with our thoughts and fears and a bunch of unanswered questions about what our partners really think and feel about us.

Hundreds, maybe thousands of times, my wife tried to communicate that something was wrong. That something hurt.

*But that doesn't make sense. I'm not trying to hurt her; therefore, she shouldn't feel hurt.*

We didn't go down in a fiery explosion. We bled out from 10,000 paper cuts.

Quietly. Slowly.

She knew something was wrong. I insisted everything was fine.

This is how your marriage ends.

*Romantic partners or spouses who*

*frequently, if not always, remember to*

*consider each other in their decision-making*

*each day are the kind of people who trust one*

*another and who trust that their partnership*

*or marriage will go the distance.*

## 2

# GOOD PEOPLE CAN BE BAD SPOUSES

MOST OF US ENTER MARRIAGE AS I IMAGINE WE WOULD ON AN
episode of the pretend television show *Marriage: Survivor Island.*

Because that's what marriage essentially is, right? No matter how
wonderful our parents and extended families are, and no matter the
quality of our education and academic experiences, marriage is essentially the equivalent of everyone we invite to our wedding being on the
same jumbo plane with us and bidding us farewell as we parachute
onto some island that we think we understand but actually know next
to nothing about.

We know how to eat and that we must. But do we know where to
find food and what on the island is safe to eat? Maybe we know how
to build a shelter. But do we know what location makes sense and what
might threaten our safety—weather, disease, animals, other people? We
kind-of, sort-of know how to not die, but in this case, we don't even
know what may or may not be fatal.

*"Good luck!!! We love you guys!!! Never go to bed angry!!!"* they all smile and wave to us and blow bubbles or throw dried rice with the best of intentions and fortune-cookie marriage advice, as they're sending us off on the ultimate Darwinian experience.

O

No one tells us the truth about marriage, and even if they try, it doesn't register because most of us don't take anything seriously that isn't an immediate threat. It's cliché but also an important truth: We don't know what we don't know.

The adults did us a disservice as we were growing up. They didn't give us the real story. They didn't give us the dirt. They didn't tell us the truth.

They didn't tell us how the things that actually destroy love and marriage disguise themselves as unimportant and inconsequential. They didn't tell us that the most dangerous things neither APPEAR nor FEEL dangerous as they're happening. They didn't warn us that the slow and steady buildup of thousands of little things—thousands of paper cuts—is what will ultimately erode any semblance of trust and intimacy and that it often results in the eventual collapse of a marriage and family.

Some of this well-intentioned deception was about protecting us, of course. If you're a parent like me, it's not difficult to empathize. The adults wanted to preserve our innocence. They wanted us to believe in Santa Claus because it was fun and made us feel happy.

We shouldn't blame our parents for our problems. Nor do I believe that my teachers or coaches or other adults in my life when I was growing up are responsible for me being a shitty husband. We all make (or don't make) the beds we sleep in.

If we lined them all up and asked them about it, we'd discover that their parents, teachers, and coaches didn't tell them any of this shit either. Everyone inherited ignorance and blindness. You can tell by looking at the putrid success rate of marriage and long-term romantic relationships.

I don't pretend to have the market cornered on marital wisdom and best practices. I'm still just some divorced asshole. I have the same questions about combating the divorce epidemic and unhealthy relationships as you.

Because this is not okay. Most people feeling extreme discontent in their most important relationships does not contribute positively to the world at large. I don't know how to measure just how much all of the interpersonal fuckery is adversely affecting us on a societal scale (think civil and political unrest), but I struggle to imagine that there are very many members of violent, angry mobs who would report high relationship satisfaction at home.

One of the ways we can make this world a better place is by getting collectively serious about educating both ourselves and younger generations about the knowledge and skills we will need to excel in our human relationships. As parents, maybe we can prepare our children in ways we were not, to navigate the emotional minefield of adult relationships—particularly long-term romantic ones like marriage. And, societally, maybe we can spend more time thinking about and talking about how to arm our students in the education system with some of this knowledge and some of these skills.

Do you want to guess how many times the Pythagorean theorem, or being able to differentiate igneous from sedimentary rock, or knowing which generals led the armies in the War of 1812 ever made a meaningful difference in my life?

I do this work because I care about everyone out there fighting their fights who don't even know what to watch out for or where to direct their energy within their relationships. I do this work to fight for all of the crying little kids who want only for Mom and Dad to love one another and keep them safe.

The state of human relationships, and the adverse effects on individuals living in them, is a global problem. One we ignore at our peril.

So, let's talk about some of the ideas that made me a better human, which might have saved my marriage, and maybe can help you or someone you love.

○

I always thought of myself as a good person. I mentioned this before because it is true and relevant to how I got into this mess.

This has been the case since my earliest memories. I knew that I loved people and hated no one. I knew that I valued concepts I associate with the idea of "being good." I knew that I'd never hurt anyone intentionally—ever—and that when it became evident to me that I HAD hurt someone, I always felt horrible about it and wished it hadn't happened.

I am not—nor have I ever been—someone who wants to harm others. And I believe (not naively, I hope) that most people are this way. That most romantic partners are this way.

This idea is important because I believed the invisible ingredients that make us who we are—that make us so-called good or bad people—were the same ingredients that determined whether I was a good husband or a bad husband. A good father or a bad father. A good friend or a bad friend.

*Because I'm a good person who loves his wife, who thinks and feels*

*good things toward her, and who would never harm her intentionally, I*
*am a good husband!*

Pretty silly, huh? Or maybe you think and feel that too.

That idea seems absurd to me today. Life offers us countless examples of lovely, amazing, admirable humans who are maybe not so good
at performing a particular function or role.

My grandmother is the sweetest, kindest person who has ever existed. Anyone who says differently is a dirty liar or possibly just someone
who has never met her. Despite my grandmother's impeccable character, I don't perceive her to be the optimum choice to pilot a race car,
to lead an architectural team to design a New York City high-rise, or to
repair your broken watch.

Skillfully driving race cars, designing buildings that won't fall down,
and fixing broken watches have very little to do with how good of a person
someone is.

Developing knowledgeable expertise on a particular subject matter
as well as mastery of skills to perform tasks at a high level requires both
study and practice. Yet many of us don't consider relationships to be
something on which we should work to develop mastery.

Imagine being in culinary school and whipping together a shitty
omelet with runny eggs, rotting vegetables, doused in rancid vinegar,
and then protesting your cooking instructor hating the food you made
on the basis that you're a well-liked person who supports local charities.

That must have been how I sounded to my wife.

My body would tense up and then I would make the incredulous
squinty-eyed, half-frowny face that I make anytime I see or hear something my brain calculates to be ridiculous. I don't think I've ever seen
exactly what I look like when I make that face, but it's fair to assume
you'd want to punch it.

When I wasn't making the punch-worthy *Everything you're saying is wrong and stupid!* face, I'd have a blank expression and stare at my wife dumbly because of the WTF out-of-body experience I was having similar to the handful of times I swallowed mushrooms in college, only minus the fun.

> WIFE: *"You just did a thing that hurt me. Not a little. A lot. It feels like you don't love me. I don't know how I'm supposed to trust you nor how I'm supposed to feel confident that we can have a peaceful, sustainable marriage when you repeatedly do or say hurtful things to me."*

> ME: *"That's silly. I would never ever want you to feel hurt; therefore, you SHOULDN'T feel hurt! I love you! I'm a nice person! People like me! You're literally the only person who ever complains about me! You treat me like I'm a bad husband, but I'm a good guy!"*

Because in my mind I was a good person, and therefore a good husband, her suggestions to the contrary were summarily dismissed as the overemotional and inaccurate accusations of an ungrateful wife who lacked perspective.

She felt unloved, she said. *Uhhh. But I literally love you more than anyone. Can't you tell by the fact that I married you and give everything I have to you and exchanged my previous fun, single life to spend the rest of my life with you?*

*Imagine being this ungrateful and tone-deaf. Dudes are out there hitting their wives, sleeping with their co-workers, committing crimes, staying out all night drinking, etc., and I'm not a good husband?!*

*I don't do all of these horrible things that bad men do—that bad husbands do! Why is she always complaining about the negative things I do without ever acknowledging any of the positives?*

I didn't figure it out until long after our marriage had ended: **Good men can be bad husbands. Good people can be bad spouses.**

But before I came to that conclusion, every suggestion that I might be hurting my wife or that I might have room for improving certain behaviors in the marriage was met with resistance.

Thankfully, I was around to explain it to her. *Once she hears this more accurate interpretation of the situation, is exposed to a more rational way of thinking and feeling about it, and has a clearer understanding of why I did what I did, everything will be fine, and we can move on! Yay for happy marriage!*

## THE INVALIDATION TRIPLE THREAT: THE LEADING CAUSE OF RELATIONSHIP FAILURE SINCE 3.5M BC

Researching the leading causes of divorce yields ambiguous answers such as "Irreconcilable differences," a "Lack of commitment," or a short and straight-to-the-point "Conflict."

Those answers are valid but about as specific as a medical examiner or coroner determining a person's cause of death to be "brain stopped functioning" or "heart quit pumping blood."

Umm. Yeah, they did. But why?

The world's leading cause of relationship failure—I believe—is a sneaky little conversation pattern in marriage and romantic relationships that I call the Invalidation Triple Threat.

You probably experience and participate in this poisonous verbal merry-go-round—as either the invalidator or the person being invalidated (perhaps you reverse roles sometimes depending on the subject matter)—and this is me asking you to kindly cut that shit out pronto.

*The Invalidation Triple Threat erodes trust every time it occurs.*

It disguises itself as harmless disagreement that's nothing for us to worry about. So, it often continues unabated, sneakily eroding trust one new paper cut at a time until no trust is left.

No trust = no relationship. It's only a matter of time.

○

**Note on sex and gender stereotypes:** Blanket statements suggesting that men do things a certain male way and that women do things in a from-another-planet female way seem irresponsible and incomplete because those stereotypes exclude a lot of people. People who don't fit neatly into these stereotypes also have marriages and families, and they experience the same thematic relationship problems—even if the details are a little different (sometimes Dad stays home with the kids and Mom is the financial breadwinner, sometimes Dad does the majority of housework and Mom is the disorganized one, sometimes both partners are the same sex, etc.). That said, I won't be able to sleep at night if I pretend as if women are not on the receiving end of this trust-eroding and relationship-ending behavior infinitely more often than men are. Sex and gender roles are a relevant part of this conversation. We'll get to that.

○

The Invalidation Triple Threat isn't just a fun name. Literally, there are **three distinct invalidating ways** in which people commonly respond to their significant others, and I submit that this toxic conversation pattern is the world's No. 1 marriage killer.

Even though this must have happened several times per week if not several times per day in my marriage, it's as if I could never see it coming.

I would be minding my own business, not hurting anyone, and not engaging in any obviously offensive behavior. Just living my life. Watching a ball game. Sitting at the dinner table. Driving in a car. Whatever. Then—boom—my wife would interrupt my comfortable state of being to introduce some negative thing that she was experiencing and was now trying to make MY problem.

Or at least that's the *My wife is freaking out over a fish sandwich again!* version of how it went down.

A more honest version is that something had happened that resulted in my wife feeling a negative emotion—often something painful. She felt hurt, or sad, or afraid, or stressed, or anxious, or frustrated, or angry. She would then attempt to communicate this negative experience to me.

My wife's objective was not to make me uncomfortable. My wife's objective was not to attack my character. My wife's objective was not to complain about what a shitty husband she might have considered me to be.

The desired outcome of this conversation for my wife was twofold:

1. Make me aware of something negative—often painful—that she had experienced or was experiencing. Something bad had just happened and she wanted to make me aware of it. How else could I know?

2. Recruit me to cooperate with her moving forward or to help her stop hurting right in that moment. If I understood how and why what had recently occurred had hurt my wife, I would be able to more effectively participate in the bad thing never happening again.

You can probably guess how often my wife's efforts to communicate and connect with me in this way were rewarded with expressed concern for her well-being or a genuine desire to change anything I was doing. *I'm not doing anything wrong! I don't try to change you! Stop trying to change me!*

### Invalidation Triple Threat Response #1:
### My Wife's Thoughts Were Wrong

Event X happened, which resulted in my wife experiencing pain or another negative emotion—anger, embarrassment, fear, sadness— anything that sucks to feel.

"Hey Matt. Event X happened, and it made me feel shitty," she said.

And I'd say, "But wait. Event X DIDN'T happen the way you're say- ing it did. You're getting the facts wrong. You shouldn't feel hurt because you're wrong about what happened. What actually happened was . . ."

The first version of the Invalidation Triple Threat involves judg- ing other people's recollection of events or their perception of reality to be fundamentally flawed. The negative feelings my wife was having should have never been happening in the first place, I reasoned.

*If the so-called painful event weren't actually painful since it didn't happen the way you said it did, then there is no longer any reason for you to feel bad about it or to continue making me responsible for your feelings! Problem solved!*

### Invalidation Triple Threat Response #2:
### My Wife's Feelings Were Wrong

Event Y happened. My wife experienced pain or another negative emotion—anger, embarrassment, fear, sadness—anything that sucks to feel.

"Hey Matt. Event Y happened, and it made me feel shitty," she said.

And I'd say, "But wait. Sure, Event Y happened, but why are you making a big deal out of it? It doesn't make sense for you to feel those feelings because of Event Y. When Event Y happens, a more normal or healthy response is to . . ."

The second version of the Invalidation Triple Threat involves judging other people's emotional experiences to be out of alignment with what we perceive to be a fair or appropriate response.

My wife's feelings were invalid because they were an overreaction (or perhaps an underreaction) to what had occurred, I figured.

My wife communicated that something had happened, and I judged her stated lived experience to be incorrect.

Her emotions were wrong.

*You're overreacting! If you recalibrate your feelings to not care so much about that, you will magically not feel bad anymore! Just like me! You should try it because MY emotions are clearly better and healthier than YOUR emotions!*

### Invalidation Triple Threat Response #3: The Justifiable Defense

This one is scary because I perceive it to be the most damaging, the most common, and—ironically—the most defensible.

Event Z happened. This time, I had directly done something or failed to do something, which resulted in my wife feeling something bad.

"Hey Matt. Event Z happened, and it made me feel shitty," she said.

And I'd say, "But wait. Let me explain!" And then proceed to make the case for how it made so much sense for me to do whatever led to Event Z.

*If you understand the situation as I understood it, you will clearly see that I'm innocent of all wrongdoing, so you shouldn't feel bad! And IF you're going to feel bad anyway, you shouldn't feel bad toward me because it was all one big misunderstanding!*

The third and most-damaging version of the Invalidation Triple Threat involves defending or explaining your actions to justify them.

It erodes trust in TWO ways. Not only does it invalidate the expressed thoughts and feelings of our spouse, who just finished her or his efforts to communicate that something painful had just happened, but it also implies that we'll repeat this pain-causing behavior in the future.

My wife would tell me that something hurtful had occurred, and now she was trying to recruit me to understand that and participate cooperatively moving forward to avoid having the painful thing happen again.

But instead of demonstrating even a sliver of empathy, remorse, or compassion, I would justify my decision-making on the merits that it made sense based on the information I had.

Just like Invalidation Triple Threat Responses #1 and #2, defending myself and justifying my actions was completely dismissive of the fact that my wife is standing right in front of me, letting me know that something painful had just happened to her. I didn't appear to care about any pain my wife was feeling anytime it was linked to something I was responsible for. I only seemed to care about her feelings when I wasn't the target of her sadness or anger.

It is both this pattern and the fear of this pattern playing out over and over again that accelerates trust erosion in our relationships.

While I explained how I was so smart and righteous to do whatever I had done, my wife was hearing me more or less promise that, in all similar future scenarios, her pain—her feelings of being loved, respected, cared for—would not matter as much to me as whatever super-smart and logical calculation I had made.

My wife, over and over again, heard me promise to hurt her again in the future. I thought I was intelligently sharing a different way to think about it so that my wife could adjust her silly feelings so she wouldn't be inconvenienced by them.

*I don't need to change because I'm a good person who didn't do anything wrong. SHE needs to change because it isn't fair that she's making her emotions MY responsibility!*

My wife was left to conclude that not only was I unconcerned with whether she felt hurt by something but that I would always choose what I wanted even when what I wanted was painful for her.

She was left to conclude that tomorrow and next month and five years from now would hurt as much or more than today. The future looked darker and threatening. Not bright nor hopeful. No matter how much she wanted it to. No matter how convinced I was that I was a good person making good choices.

○

The Invalidation Triple Threat DAMAGES people. It triggers conflict and erodes trust just a little bit more every time it happens, and holy shit does it happen often.

You don't need to be evil or ill-intentioned to engage in these marriage-killing conversations. We can participate in these conversations with total integrity—feeling love in our hearts and while telling no lies.

Good people telling the truth as they see it. Do you see the problem? THAT is how marriages get destroyed.

A well-intentioned spouse who loves his or her partner can—with honesty and integrity—disagree with someone's account of what just happened. *Wait. I think you're making an honest mistake. Here's what really happened.*

A well-intentioned spouse can lovingly and honestly believe that his or her spouse is feeling negative emotions unnecessarily. *Wait. I love you and I don't want you to feel these horrible things. Is it possible that this is beneath you? That you're allowing something insignificant to have more power over your life than it should?*

And a loving, honest spouse can have a totally legitimate reason to have made his or her decision that resulted in this painful experience. *If you'll let me explain what I knew at the time, I think you'll see that you would have made the same decisions that I did!*

The Invalidation Triple Threat doesn't look scary. It sounds like two people who love each other having a harmless disagreement. *No big deal!*

And yet it happens over and over and over again. Several times per day. Sometimes, several times during the same conversation. Each time, a little bit of trust disappears. A little bit more safety disappears.

It's the beginning of the slow march toward the end of our relationship, and we have no idea that's what's happening or just how uncomfortable it's going to become down the road.

## SHE DIVORCED ME BECAUSE I LEFT DISHES BY THE SINK

In January 2016, I published a blog post with the title "She Divorced Me Because I Left Dishes by the Sink." I didn't set out to write a gimmicky, click-bait article. It was simply my next attempt to leverage personal stories and my affinity for metaphor to share ideas about what I had come to believe harms marriages.

A week after publishing it, several million people had read it, and it remains the most popular and most-shared thing I've ever written. Some readers called me an idiot. Others thanked me for saving their marriage.

Here's the new, improved, and updated version without the whole Men Always Do Things This Way and Women Always Do Things This Other Way vibe. (Because that's not how it works.)

○

It seems so unreasonable when you put it that way: *My wife left me because sometimes I leave dishes by the sink.*

It makes her seem ridiculous and makes me seem like a victim of unfair expectations.

We like to point fingers at other things to explain why something went wrong, like when Biff Tannen crashed George McFly's car and spilled beer on his clothes, but it was all George's fault for not telling him the car had a blind spot.

*This bad thing happened because of this, that, and the other thing. Not because of anything I did!*

Sometimes I leave used drinking glasses by the kitchen sink, just inches away from the dishwasher. It isn't a big deal to me now. It wasn't a big deal to me when I was married. But it WAS a big deal to her.

Each time my wife entered the kitchen to discover the glass I'd left next to the sink, she moved incrementally closer to moving out and ending our marriage. I just didn't know it yet. But even if I had, I fear I wouldn't have worked as hard to change my behavior as I would have stubbornly tried to get her to see things my way.

I think that I believed my wife should respect me simply because I exchanged vows with her. It wouldn't have been the first time I acted entitled. What I know for sure is that I never connected putting a dish in the dishwasher with earning my wife's respect.

I remember my wife saying how exhausting it was for her to have to tell me what to do all the time. It's why one of the sexiest things we can say to our partner is "I got this," and then take care of whatever needs taken care of. (Or perhaps take care of it without announcing it or seeking praise for having contributed meaningfully to our shared home lives.)

I always reasoned, "If you just tell me what you want me to do, I'll gladly do it."

But my wife didn't want to be my mother. She wanted to be my adult partner, and she wanted me to apply all of my intelligence and learning capabilities to the logistics of managing our lives and household.

She wanted me to figure out what needed to be done in order for our lives to function effectively, and then devise my own method of task management without making her responsible for orchestrating everything.

I wish I could remember what seemed so unreasonable to me about that at the time.

## MEN CAN DO THINGS!

We'll dive into so-called traditional gender roles later and discuss how they influence the quality of our relationships, but for now let's just say that I passively stood to the side in my marriage in regard to shared domestic duties, and even more egregiously, when it came to bringing our baby home and raising a child together. If I didn't feel confident that I could perform a task or develop a system as effectively as my wife, I would simply check out of the process entirely, trusting that she would find a way. I was right to defer to her because she was amazing at those things, but I was wrong to run away from shared responsibilities and was blind to the pain caused by abandoning our spouses to manage households, children, and other aspects of marriage alone.

Maybe my assessment that I was ill-equipped to perform certain domestic duties was spot-on. But the answer was not to check out, forcing my wife to do everything, but rather to expand my knowledge base and skill set to eliminate whatever I was missing.

Change is uncomfortable. Learning new things is hard. So, I chose comfort, which forced my wife to carry the uncomfortable parts of marriage and child-rearing alone.

In the back of my mind, the thought was always there: *I'm a guy. She's a woman. She's good at this stuff. I'm not. Therefore, she can handle it and I should just stay out of her way.*

O

Men, it turns out, invented heavy machines that can fly in the air reliably and safely. Men proved the heliocentric model of the solar system, establishing that the earth orbits the sun.

Today, men are seen designing and building skyscrapers. We see other men taking human organs out of dead people and using them to replace failing organs from inside of living people who need them. And then those people stay alive after. Which is insane.

The point? Men are totally good at stuff when they try hard.

I was perfectly capable of doing many of the things I abandoned my wife to do alone.

You may be wondering, *"Hey Matt! Why would you leave a glass by the sink instead of putting it in the dishwasher?!"*

Several reasons:

1. I may want to use it again.

2. I—personally—don't care if a glass is sitting by the sink unless guests are visiting.

3. I will never care about a glass sitting by the sink. Ever. It's impossible. It's like asking me to make myself interested in crocheting or to enjoy yard work. I don't want to crochet things. And it's hard for me to imagine a scenario in which working in my yard sounds more appealing than any of several thousand less-sucky things that could be done instead.

There is only one reason I will ever stop leaving that glass by the sink, and it's a lesson I learned much too late: because I love and respect my partner, and it really matters to them.

I now understand that when I left that glass there, it hurt my wife—literally causing pain—because it felt to her as if I had just said, "Hey. I don't respect you or value your thoughts and opinions. Not taking four seconds to put my glass in the dishwasher is more important to me than you are."

Suddenly, this moment is no longer about something as benign and meaningless as a dirty dish.

Now, this moment is about a meaningful act of love and sacrifice.

It occurred to me later that I didn't have to understand WHY my wife cared about the things that she did. (Though I think digging for that "why" is always a worthwhile exercise.)

The only thing I needed to understand was that my wife did care. I needed to understand what was important to her and what was not important to her. And then demonstrate respect for things on her This Is Important to Me list.

Then maybe I would have figured out before it was too late that me loving my wife in my brain and feeling love for my wife in my chest wasn't nearly as important as conveying that idea through acts of love.

Just as good people with good intentions can speak and act in a manner that accidentally results in harm (such as offering a peanut butter cookie to someone with a fatal nut allergy), people who honestly love someone can inadvertently communicate something else.

By understanding that my wife experienced meaningful pain—just like all of the unpleasant shit I feel when things hurt me—from something like this glass sitting next to the sink, I could have communicated my love and respect for her by NOT leaving tiny reminders for her each day that she wasn't considered. That she wasn't remembered. That she wasn't respected. I could have carefully avoided leaving evidence that I would always choose my feelings and my preferences over hers.

Then, caring about her = putting glass in the dishwasher.

Caring about her = keeping your laundry off the floor.

Caring about her = thoughtfully not tracking dirt or whatever on the floor she worked hard to clean.

Caring about her = taking care of kid-related things so she can just chill out for a little bit and worry about one less thing.

Caring about her = "Hey babe. Is there anything I can do today or pick up on my way home that will make your day better?"

Caring about her = a million little things that say "I love you" more than speaking the words ever could.

○

It's not easy. But it might be that simple. People capable of those mental and behavioral changes can have a great relationship.

It's as if we want to fight for our right to leave that glass there. Because maybe we don't think it's fair that our partner's preferences should always win out over ours.

It might look like this:

*Eat shit, wife, we think. I sacrifice a lot for you, and you're going to get on me about ONE glass by the sink? THAT little bullshit glass that takes a few seconds to put in the dishwasher, which I'll gladly do when I know I'm done with it, is so important to you that you want to give me crap about it? You want to take an otherwise peaceful evening and have an argument with me, and tell me how I'm getting something wrong and failing you, over this glass? After all of the big things I do to make our life possible—things I never hear a 'thank you' for (and don't ask for)—you're going to elevate a glass by the sink into a marriage problem? I couldn't be THAT petty if I tried. And I need to dig my heels in on this one. If you want that glass in the dishwasher, put it in there yourself without telling me about it. Otherwise, I'll put it away when people are coming over, or when I'm done with it. This is a bullshit fight that feels unfair and I'm not just going to bend over for you.*

I wanted my wife to agree that when you put life in perspective, a drinking glass by the sink that no one but us will ever see, and the solution taking all of four seconds, is simply not a big problem that should cause a marriage fight.

I thought she should recognize how petty and meaningless it was in the grand scheme of life. I repeated that train of thought for the better part of twelve years, waiting for her to finally agree with me.

But she never did. She never agreed.

I was arguing about the merits of a glass by the sink. But for my wife, it wasn't about the glass. It wasn't about dishes by the sink, or laundry on the floor, or her trying to get out of doing the work of caring for our son for whom there's nothing she wouldn't do.

It was about this idea of consideration. About the pervasive sense that she was married to someone who did not respect nor appreciate her. And if I didn't respect or appreciate her, then I didn't love her in a manner that felt trustworthy.

She couldn't count on the adult who had promised to love her forever because none of this dish-by-the-sink business felt anything like being loved.

When there's no trust, there can be no safety. People who do not feel safe will always seek safety. In marriage, that means our partners must leave us and find a new living arrangement that brings about security and contentment. Conditions in which pain is not the daily experience.

If I knew that this drinking glass situation and similar arguments are what would actually end my marriage—that the existence of love and trust and respect and safety existing in our marriage were dependent on these moments I was writing off as petty disagreements, I would have made different choices.

"*I never get upset with you about things you do that I don't like!*" I reasoned, as if my wife were intentionally choosing to feel hurt and miserable.

When you choose to love someone, it becomes your pleasure to do things that enhance their lives and bring you closer together, rather than a chore.

It's not: *Sonofabitch, I have to do this bullshit thing for my wife again.*

It's: *I'm grateful for another opportunity to demonstrate to my wife that she comes first and that I can be counted on to be there for her and that she needn't look elsewhere for happiness and fulfillment.*

Once I learned how to equate this glass situation about which I didn't feel emotion with an action that DID inflict pain on my wife and damaged my marriage, I transformed from someone who was a perpetual threat into someone who wasn't.

Of course, this realization occurred years after our marriage ended. It would have been neat to understand these ideas much sooner.

## FOR YOUR CONSIDERATION: HOW OFTEN DO YOU REMEMBER YOUR SPOUSE WHEN YOU MAKE DECISIONS?

The reasons more than half of all romantic relationships (including marriage) fail are not obvious to most people.

If you need proof, just ask your current or former relationship partner to share their beliefs about what you experience—good and bad—in your relationship (or your reasons for wanting to leave your former partner).

I'm willing to bet that eight—probably nine—times out of ten, their answer will fall well short of accurately describing your experiences, highlighting all of the ways they don't quite understand what matters to you, and what doesn't.

Unless you can tell the story of your marriage (or any romantic relationship) challenges in a way that results in your partner nodding their head and saying, "Yes. That is exactly right. That is exactly how I feel," then you can safely dismiss the idea that you know and understand your partner well enough to avoid conflict and communicate effectively.

○

*"I want to feel like the person I married considers me when they make decisions,"* many wives and a handful of husbands have said to me.

I frequently did not consider how my decisions, words, and actions affected my wife, and after several painful years of being on the receiving end of that lack of consideration, she chose to leave.

Sometimes I'd leave a pair of jeans on a piece of furniture in our bedroom. Jeans that weren't dirty enough to throw in the laundry. She hated it and asked me not to. I treated her as if she were wrong or crazy for always needing her preferences to win over mine.

Other times I would make jokes at her expense in front of our friends and then defend it because I wasn't trying to hurt her feelings. I treated her as if she was emotionally weak when she would mention it later. As if she were wrong or crazy for reacting to what I perceived to be harmless, playful jokes.

She spoke up. I didn't listen. She experienced me as either not believing her claims of feeling pain from situations like this or perhaps as me not giving a shit regardless.

My wife was married to a man who frequently made decisions that would directly or inadvertently affect her—sometimes in substantially negative ways. And my defense was that it was an accident. That I didn't mean to. I fought for that recognition. I really believed that things were never as bad as she made them out to be. *I'm a good guy! I seriously love you! I'm NEVER trying to hurt or upset you!*

She always acted as if that didn't matter, and I always acted as if she were being unfair. I spent our entire relationship missing the point.

It's not that I considered my wife and then made a bunch of decisions that hurt or inconvenienced or disrespected her afterward.

The more significant idea is that I often went about my days never considering her at all. **I frequently made decisions in which my wife was not a factor in the math equation my brain used to decide something.**

THAT is what hurts the people we love. Not that we're a bunch of assholes doing a bunch of asshole things on purpose to sabotage our marriages. Of course, we're not doing that.

The idea that creates intense pain and erodes trust in our relationships is what my wife experienced as being so seemingly inconsequential to me—so unworthy of my care and concern—that I would blindly or thoughtlessly make decisions without factoring in how she might be affected by them.

It didn't occur to me to ask my wife how she might feel about it or to spend any time considering it.

I was often perplexed—even offended—by her making a big deal out of whatever new little thing had been needlessly elevated to a marriage problem. I was so focused on my disappointment in what I perceived to be a never-ending stream of new complaints about me that I didn't recognize the idea that would have saved my marriage and family.

My wife's aim was NOT to complain about me or attack my character, though I usually responded in a defensive, invalidating manner indicating that I thought that's what she was unfairly doing.

She wanted to feel loved. Cherished. Respected. Desired.

My wife wanted her husband to think and act as if she were worthy of being considered—that she was important enough for me to remember, and respect, and think about when I was making decisions, no matter how inconsequential I might have believed these decisions to be.

Romantic partners or spouses who frequently, if not always, remember to consider each other in their decision-making each day are the kind of people who trust one another and who trust that their partnership or marriage will go the distance.

And as we will discuss next, the quality of your relationship and its capacity for withstanding the ups and downs that adult life delivers will be influenced most greatly by the amount of trust you and your partner build and maintain with each other.

*But then we wake up as adults and, sooner or later, must face the truth—our feelings matter. They do.*

3

# THE INVALIDATION TRIPLE THREAT: THE DANGER HIDING IN THE SHADOWS

**SAFE**–adj.–\'sāf\—secure from threat of danger, harm, or loss

**TRUST**–verb–\'trəst\—to commit or place in one's care or keeping; to place confidence in, rely on; to hope or expect confidently

O

"You don't make me feel safe," my wife said. "I don't feel like I can trust you anymore."

*That's absurd*, I thought.

My concept of safety was rooted in the idea of physical safety. Wearing a seat belt. Not getting pistol-whipped during an armed robbery. Wearing the proper safety equipment on a construction site or in a manufacturing facility or during a football or baseball game.

In relationship terms, I thought about the idea of safety in the context of protecting my wife from physical harm.

*I want to sleep closest to the bedroom door.*

*I want to be the one to check out the strange noise in the house.*

*I want to be with her walking in a dimly lit parking garage at night.*

*I want to pay for a home-security system to deter and warn of intruders.*

*I want to fight and take the potential beatdown to give her time to run away.*

*I want to take the bullet for her.*

*And I will never physically harm her. Ever.*

And because of those things, I thought my wife (and anyone, really) should feel safe with me. I thought those things made me a person who was safe to be with.

O

Safety is probably more important to you than you consciously realize in any given moment. After basic metabolic functions like breathing and heartbeats, as well as survival basics (food, water, shelter, and clothing), safety is next on the list of things living creatures require.

People need things.

We can debate semantics surrounding the word "need," like whether electricity or indoor plumbing or Wi-Fi or sex or vehicles qualify. But if you will grant me some latitude on the verbiage, it will help.

Psychologist Abraham Maslow famously published his hierarchy of needs in 1943. The idea is that once we satisfy the most basic level of human need, we can advance to the next one, and then the next, until we reach the pinnacle of living our best lives.

It is commonly presented in pyramid form like this:

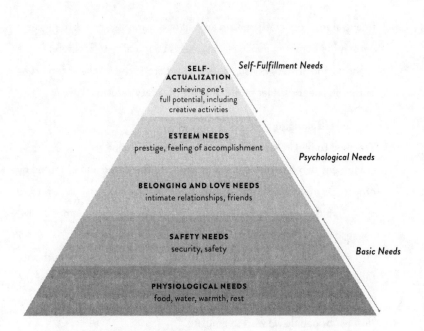

In reverse pyramid-stacking order, people need:

1. **Physiological (or Basic) Needs**

We need air, water, food, clothes, and shelter. Typically, if any of those are missing, we don't care about things we might normally care about, like family drama, the economy, or the season finale of our favorite television show.

2. **Safety**

We need to feel safe.

If lions and bears are chasing us, or if we have a gun pointed at us, or if we are diagnosed with a life-changing or threatening disease, or if the financial markets crash and we lose all of our money, or if bad guys are detonating bombs in public places, we lose our ability to feel safe.

Stress and anxiety consume us, and we are stuck on the second rung of this life-needs ladder until our sense of safety returns.

### 3.  Love/Belonging

We need to feel loved and/or as if we belong to a tribe.

Humans demonstrate a profound need to feel loved and accepted by others. So much so that we sometimes sacrifice our personal safety to cling to abusive people (physically, sexually, mentally, and/or emotionally) because of how much we crave their love and acceptance.

These people can be romantic partners, parents, caregivers, authority figures, or people we believe are our friends. We do this in pursuit of the feeling of being loved by, and connected to, others we identify as being "like us" or people we wish to emulate.

### 4.  Esteem

We need to feel respected and accepted.

We crave professional success, mastery of a hobby, accumulation of wealth, and victory in competition. Many people crave fame and recognition in pursuit of feeling respected by others, though it doesn't have to be as gross as that might sound. Maybe, for example, you're a middle-aged, divorced, single father who is so ashamed of your failings as a husband and dad that you withdraw from most of your friends and family and mostly hide from the world. But then, miraculously, you're given an opportunity to be a fancy book author and you feel slightly less pathetic and broken, so maybe you won't skip the next high school class reunion like you have in the past.

Maslow called this craving for the approval of others the Lower form of Esteem. Leveraging others' opinions as evidence that we are good enough. Checks out.

He called it the Lower form of Esteem because we can never legitimately feel respected and accepted until we decide to respect and accept ourselves. Self-respect, Maslow said, is the Higher form of Esteem.

5. **Self-Actualization/Transcendence**

We need to achieve whatever our individual or collective potential is and accomplish whatever we are capable of to live and die without shame or regret. This is the Higher form of Esteem. When we feel the gratification of having value, not from how we think others perceive us, but that we generate ourselves.

Psychology teaches us that feelings of self-loathing or as if we're not good enough poison our relationships, sometimes causing us to underestimate a partner's love. Poor self-esteem can result in us interpreting our partner's actions in the most negative terms possible because we subconsciously question whether we're worthy of their love. This condition results in feelings of anxiety and the expectation of rejection, the result of which is us interpreting neutral or benign actions as rejecting or "mean."

Mental health professionals advocate healthy self-love, which is best described as self-acceptance. To believe yourself to be worthy of being loved, without having to prove yourself to other people. When we love and accept ourselves, we are less likely to exhibit burdensome neediness to our romantic partner (or anyone we love) by showing up as excessively critical of their behavior, or by demanding excessive reassurance from them.

As you move up the five-step pyramid from Basic Needs for staying alive to more mind- and heart-based needs, you will notice the pyramid levels—and the number of people who have achieved them—getting smaller and smaller.

That is because we must not only understand but also master a human need before we are able to ascend to the next level.

Some people, for many reasons, live entire lives without feeling loved, without respecting themselves, and never really feeling safe or comfortable in their own skin.

Let the record show you can also regress and fall down a peg or two.

I've lived many years succeeding in the #4 Esteem space, but now I mostly stumble around back down in #2 (an apt bathroom metaphor), trying to figure out what the hell is wrong with me and whether I'm even capable of pulling myself out of the post-divorce morass and achieving a satisfying life for myself and those I love.

O

*"Hey Matt! Is my relationship suffering because my partner's or my own literal needs aren't being met?"*

Yep.

You need things. And your partner does too. And when one or both of you need things, you will (often involuntarily) pursue them.

And the simple truth is this: **When we are obstacles to our partners' pursuit of their own needs, or when we neglect to fulfill any needs that fall to us as their partners, we are complicit in their decisions to pursue those needs elsewhere.**

That doesn't mean it's cool to cheat on your partner because they won't agree to threesomes or to get yourself off looking at internet porn at the expense of sex with your spouse because you claim they don't satisfy your superficial sexual "needs."

Nor does it mean it's suddenly cool to have an affair with Heidi from work or Brad from the gym because the attention they provide strokes your lovey-dovey, feel-good emotional needs.

But it DOES mean that we should all be super-intentional about discovering our partner's needs (not what WE think they are, but what THEY know they are) and commit to helping them achieve their personal five levels of the human-needs pyramid and become their best-possible selves.

Either that or communicate honestly and clearly that we are unwilling to so that they can then pursue a life without us deliberately holding them down.

Not supporting our partner's pursuit of living their best life does not justify them betraying or abusing us. But does it justify them choosing a life in which we are no longer the obstacle in their way because we are unwilling or unable to move?

Decide for yourself. My wife left. When it happened, I thought she was mistreating me, and I cried and yelled and blamed her for ruining my life. Today, I believe she made a wise choice given her circumstances and data set from our prior twelve years together. When someone feels perpetually mistreated and unloved, it's both sensible and healthy for them to consider whether voluntarily choosing that every day forever is the right thing to do.

In the same way that individuals are stuck on a certain level of the hierarchy of needs pyramid until they've fulfilled a specific need, our relationships get stuck on those same levels—often Level 2. When there is no trust, there is no safety, and when there is no safety, then we cannot connect with one another on the Love & Belonging, or Esteem, levels.

Have you ever offered a gift, kind words, a show of physical affection, or demonstrated sexual desire for your romantic partner, only to have those actions rebuffed somehow, resulting in feelings of rejection?

People often get upset when this happens. In both my experience as a relationship coach and my own personal experience, men are more reactive and sensitive to this form of being refused.

*"She says she wants all of these things from me, and then when I actually try to do them, she rejects me and treats me like her enemy! No one makes me feel as unappreciated and rejected as my wife can!"*

This is NOT rejection.

This is the result of unmet needs further down the pyramid. Expensive gifts, flirty texts, and earnest efforts to contribute more around the house do not feel like thoughtful acts of love and intimacy when they are coming from the same person who triggers feelings of mistrust and a lack of safety.

People who are in the so-called doghouse in their relationships often never find their way out. We promise to change, and we seem to believe that offering flower bouquets, jewelry, vacations, date nights, and other such thoughtful acts of love and interest in our partners is the path back to their hearts.

Those may all be useful ways of communicating love and connectedness when Safety and Trust are present in the relationship, but you will find they mostly prove useless when Safety and Trust are absent.

## RELATIONSHIPS WITHER AND DIE BECAUSE PARTNERS DON'T TRUST EACH OTHER

When I was married, I honed in on the concept of infidelity when thinking about the word "trust" in relationships.

That is an understandably big deal to most people. To be loyal and trustworthy. We also seek "trustworthy" financial partners and co-parents.

I figured *I don't cheat, I don't physically abuse, I don't gamble away our living-expense money, I'm not an addict, and I'm not a threat to abandon her or our children. I'm trustworthy!*

But that is not the equation for Trust. The equation is: **Safety + Belonging + Mattering = TRUST**

That's according to author and entrepreneur Christine Comaford, who writes about neuroscience and business leadership.

There is a problem, of course: our faulty brains.

While amazing and miraculous, they are also totally unreliable. If we bought our brains at The Brain Store, most of us would have returned them already for ones we hoped would work better. (Not that I would remember where I stashed the receipt.)

Comaford counsels business executives on how to discover and fulfill employee needs in the workplace. Fundamental, primitive needs. And no matter how unimpressed an employer may be with those "needs," a failure to help employees achieve them (at home for personal reasons or at work for professional ones) will result in employees and business teams underperforming or motivating them to seek work-oriented need fulfillment elsewhere.

The parallels to our marriages and personal relationships are obvious.

○

At no point in my upbringing was I exposed to other ways of thinking about safety or taught the importance of making one's spouse feel safe and secure in these more nuanced ways.

Other safety and security needs people have in addition to not being hurt or killed in accidents or acts of violence include:

- Financial security
- Health and well-being (mental and emotional safety)

Everyone has different thresholds for what financial security looks like. Having enough money to pay for one's family's needs is a concept most mature adults understand. Even the formerly married me.

But regarding mental and emotional safety? I failed as badly as someone claiming ignorance can.

I was mentally and emotionally abusive to my wife without realizing it because if I'm not careful, I can demonstrate epic levels of self-centeredness. *Everything that happens to me, and everything I think and feel and want and believe are the truest, most important things in the world! Me me me me meeeeeeeeeeee!!!*

(I'm getting a lot better. I promise.)

But I'm not the only one who seems to forget that they are not the center of the universe and that there are, in fact, about eight billion other living, breathing, thinking, feeling humans who also experience life in the same first-person way that you and I do. Only they might have different individual wants and needs, and all of those wants and needs totally make sense when you are them and not you.

## WHY COUPLES ALWAYS HAVE THE SAME FIGHT

Again, in male-female relationships (and with many same-sex couples as well), what usually happens is that two perfectly cool, sane, healthy, decent people get married—probably a little sooner than they should—while both innocently and naively believe it's always going to feel just like it does right now. *It's basically like being Forever Boyfriend and Girlfriend! We can do that!*

They love one another. They pledge faithfulness genuinely. They exchange wedding vows with the best of intentions.

And then, like clockwork, more than half of them are totally miserable within five to seven years. One or both are having affairs, or at least thinking about it, because *"they just want to feel something again!"*

He's jerking off in the shower or to late-night internet porn instead of having sex with her. She's crushing on pretty much any non-creepy guy paying attention to her and making her feel special because her husband never makes her feel important anymore.

They'll eventually divorce, or possibly stay together "for the kids" in silent misery, ensuring that pretty much every day is shitty for the rest of their lives.

Every couple has their own unique version of The Same Fight. The details vary from relationship to relationship, but the conflict pattern is virtually identical in every relationship in which trust is no longer present.

It could be any number of things. Leaving dishes in the sink. Throwing laundry on the floor. Tracking mud through the house right after your partner cleaned the floor. It doesn't matter what the actual thing is.

In the case of my client Tara, who struggles with ADHD, a common conflict trigger in her relationship revolves around time management and her propensity for tardiness. Tara's partner experiences this as disrespect—*She either can't or won't adjust her routine to be on time; I can't count on her*—and that, of course, erodes trust.

It eliminates safety. Not in a way that feels physically dangerous but in a way that feels unreliable or unsustainable in the long term.

We're always trying to reacquire that feeling of safety on the second level of Maslow's pyramid. And in the context of our relationships, the absence of reliable respect and support from our partner threatens the long-term viability of our lives together.

When Tara's partner, Miranda, shares how she feels, Tara—like so many of us—tends to fall into some form of the Invalidation Triple Threat response pattern. Usually defensiveness, she says.

What matters is that for the rest of the conversation, neither person is talking about the same thing. Tara feels hurt because the circumstances of any specific instance of tardiness was caused by some external factor—often something related to the care of their youngest child, a toddler. It doesn't seem fair to her in the moment that Miranda is making as big of a deal about it as she is.

And, of course, Tara's partner doesn't feel hurt or angry because of the one isolated incident. She is hurt and angry because it seems as if Tara doesn't love or respect her enough to be somewhere when she was supposed to be, or when she promised to be. Not the one time. Dozens of times. Hundreds of times.

In a conversation with my wife about the dish by the sink, I would think, "*What kind of insane person would want to have a horrible fight and ruin our night and make our marriage out to be a train wreck over something as insignificant as laundry or a dirty dish? I am never this irrational! If she thinks laundry and dishes are more important than our marriage, her priorities are warped, and she must not love me.*"

And my wife, much like Tara's partner, would think, "*I cannot trust this man. I can't count on him. He does NOT respect me. He never apologizes for hurting me because he doesn't think it's a big deal. He always tells me how what I think and feel is wrong or dumb. I have all these feelings and I know I'm not crazy, but he NEVER acknowledges them as important or worth his attention. He thinks 'proving' his point and winning our arguments are more important than my feelings. He doesn't care. He must not love me."*

After The Same Fight happens several hundreds of times, people stop putting as much effort into their marriage, which feels like a poor, failed, painful, unrewarding investment.

A marriage can survive on life support for a while, with just one person making a go of it. But once both quit, the relationship is effectively over. Most of us just aren't strong enough to handle the mental and emotional anguish we feel when our marriages fall apart. Nothing in our lives up to that point could have prepared us for it. Everything feels new and terrifying, and there's no instruction manual for what to do next.

The marriage breaks down imperceptibly slow—especially to a partner who honestly believes that their problems are nothing more than petty fights over arrival times or dirty dishes by the sink.

That person (which tends to be the guy in hetero couples) is liable to be blindsided by the news she's unhappy and contemplating divorce.

His wife feels as if she has been really clear about her feelings up to this point. Yet maybe her husband is like, *"What the wha-?! Why didn't you say anything?!"*

She thinks he's dumb and oblivious and disengaged. He thinks she has gone off the emotional deep end once again.

My wife knew I was reasonably smart, so she couldn't figure out how I could be so dense after hundreds of these conversations. She began to question whether I was intentionally trying to hurt her and whether I actually loved her at all.

When we're having The Same Fight, positive intent or putting up a character defense by chalking up any harm caused as accidental can be just as much of a trust killer as more overtly harmful actions.

When something damaging and painful happens because of someone else's actions, our capacity for trusting that person takes a hit. If Roger gets hammered at the local pub, hops into his pickup, and accidentally hurts or kills people in an accident after blacking out on the drive home, we might trust him less than we did before.

If Linda gets strung out on crystal meth, loses her job, and starts stealing money and valuables from family and friends to fund her addiction, we are probably going to trust her less even though her intent was not to harm the people who care for her most.

It doesn't matter whether we are intentionally refusing to cooperate with our spouses or legitimately unable to understand what's wrong—the math results are the same. The net result of The Same Fight is MORE pain. LESS trust. Regardless of anyone's intentions.

This is how two well-intentioned people slowly fall apart.

Turns out, many people don't know it. Since the only consciousness we truly understand is our individual first-person experience, it's as if many of us assume everyone else should see, think, and feel the same things that we do. We enter committed romantic relationships, including marriage, unaware that our core beliefs will inadvertently yield relationship conflict so painful and stressful that there will be days we'll want to drink ourselves into euphoric oblivion and/or launch ourselves on a space rocket and fly into the sun.

Our parents never told us otherwise, probably because they didn't want us to know how many times they almost divorced or wanted to have sex with someone else. No one explains any of this to us in school because our education officials evidently think that obtuse triangles, *The Grapes of Wrath* book reports, and pedantic lessons on the French and Indian War are more important than the information young people require to participate effectively in functional adult relationships.

Here's the thing. A dish by the sink in no way feels painful or disrespectful to a spouse who wakes up every day and experiences a marriage partner who communicates in both word and action how important and cherished their spouse and relationship are. My wife didn't flip shit over a dish by the sink because she's some insufferable nag who had to have her way all of the time. My wife communicated pain and frustration over the frequent reminders she encountered that told her over and over and over again just how little she was considered when I made decisions.

Someone else's spouse might say:

*"Because it proves you don't love me or respect me, and I don't have time to do all the laundry AND take care of everything for the kids because Kyle has a field trip Thursday and Valerie needs to get to her swim meet, and it hurts so much that I can't count on you to make sure Kyle's lunch is packed and outfit is washed and permission slip is signed, and tomorrow is the four-year anniversary of my dad dying, and—yes asshole—it still hurts, because he was the person who always made sure I was taken care of, and then I trusted you to be that person for the rest of my life, and you don't do it, and now he's gone, and just fuck you for leaving me alone in my marriage."*

O

The most common story of failing relationships involves a wife or girlfriend who loses trust in her husband or boyfriend after repeated attempts to explain why something hurts and asks for help. But none of the requests for help result in positive outcomes or evidence that he's willing to cooperate in stopping the painful behavior.

Faced with feeling hurt every day for the rest of her marriage/relationship, and no evidence her committed partner is willing to participate in making something painful go away, she stops trusting him.

No matter how good he may be. No matter how perfect his record might be in every other part of his life.

Something hurts and he either can't or won't help. She knows the relationship is unsustainable without trust. Its future is in doubt. Her security and well-being as well as that of any children they might have are now in jeopardy.

Thus, she doesn't feel safe.

And no matter how much he tries or wants to, a man she can't trust to not hurt her can't make her feel safe.

I used to believe the scariest guys in relationships were the obvious assholes. You know, the bad boys who take their no-fucks-given machismo a few toxic steps further. The guys who punch and cheat and name-call. The drunks and addicts and criminals.

But I no longer believe that because red flags are easy enough to spot. Red flags are obvious warning signs that alert people who want to steer clear.

Real danger is what lurks undetected.

You know, the "good guys." Nice. Friendly. Smart. Successful. By all appearances, good men, and good fathers.

Guys just like me.

Because when people want to end a marriage with a guy like that, you often find less support, less understanding, more disapproval, and more judgment.

*"Are you sure you're doing the right thing?! He's so nice! You're so lucky!"*

When my wife felt more afraid for her and our son than at any time in her life prior because she sensed the end coming, and perhaps—like me—felt a little guilty or ashamed for not being able to make it work, maybe what she wanted and needed most was support from those who loved her.

And the one person who had promised to love and support her forever was actually the biggest source of her pain, fear, and anxiety.

Mistrust. Unsafe. Fight or flight? She had already spent years fighting, so I left her with only one choice: *Run.*

## NOTHING IN LIFE WILL AFFECT YOU AS MUCH AS YOUR CLOSEST RELATIONSHIPS

If there's one massive gap in our formal education—or major oversight in our prioritization—I'd say we are inadvertently failing our youth by not better attempting to educate them about relationships and arming them with skills required to navigate them effectively.

We do a decent job of preparing them to get jobs in their individual areas of strength so they can make money, pay taxes, and buy stuff, but I don't think many kids graduate from any elementary, middle, or high school or school of higher education fully aware that none of their academic or professional success can save them from the horrors of crying and vomiting and seriously questioning how much they want to wake up tomorrow morning after feeling their hearts ripped out by the end of a meaningful relationship.

We were not taught nor are we teaching our kids the truth that nothing in life will affect us as profoundly as our closest interpersonal relationships—namely, marriage or a romantic relationship that looks and feels like marriage.

I mean, your health is a big deal certainly, but there is no shortage of studies linking good health to quality, connected relationships—

particularly marriage. With men, for example, marriage has been shown to actually help men live longer. And divorce is linked with all sorts of shitty things, like depression, heart disease, cancer, loneliness, etc.

This phenomenon isn't true for women. Single women tend to live longer than married women, and I'm not afraid to speculate that the reason is because many of these single women who outlived their married counterparts took action to leave dissatisfying, soul-sucking relationships. Women who labor over an unequal share of domestic responsibilities such as cleaning, cooking, shopping, laundry, raising children, caring for pets, and several more tedious, unpleasant aggravations.

Loneliness strips men of purpose and kills them faster than married or romantically partnered men.

And shitty, suffocating marriages in which they feel perpetually lonely and abandoned WITHIN the relationship kill women faster than independent women who escaped with their lives.

From an education and pre-marriage standpoint the mission, while difficult certainly, isn't complicated. We must arm boys with the knowledge and life skills necessary to avoid creating the conditions that commonly result in their partners wanting to end unhealthy relationships. (Statistically, women initiate 70 percent of divorces—often for the aforementioned reasons.)

And we must raise our girls to identify healthy relationship boundaries and communication techniques that preemptively protect themselves from getting in too deep with a partner whose behavior, over time, will erode trust to the point where they can no longer have a nontoxic, sustainable relationship or marriage.

As inconvenient as this truth is, our guiding light on this journey will be a fickle and ever-changing part of the human condition—our emotions.

# FEELINGS MATTER WHETHER OR NOT WE WANT THEM TO

This was an unpopular idea with the twentysomething version of me. *How I feel today is not necessarily how I will feel tomorrow. Sometimes I feel angry about someone or something, but after a good night's sleep that often goes away. Sometimes I feel like being alone but other times I want to be with people. Sometimes I feel like listening to rap and other times I feel like listening to guitar rock. Because feelings are ever-changing, they can't be what I use to guide my decisions. I'm going to be bigger and better and stronger than that!*

But then we wake up as adults and, sooner or later, must face the truth—our feelings matter. They do.

I spent much of my professional life working in marketing. It was in marketing that I learned that the greatest influencer of our decision-making, including what to buy at a retail store or internet website, is not our logical, reasoning mind but rather our emotional impulses.

We like to believe that we let our brains handle most of the decision-making in our lives. But nope. We do the stuff we want to do because we feel like it. Because doing so, somehow, someway, scratches an emotional itch we are having. And, of course, we avoid doing things we don't feel like doing.

Sailing the seas of life, our brains are actively influencing our choices like a nerdy, oft-disrespected and ignored first mate, but our emotion-driven bodies are rum-drunkenly piloting this vessel. *Arrrrggghhh, go fuck ye self, brain!*

If we're going to practice effective self-care so that we are healthy enough to navigate life without sabotaging ourselves or the people in our personal sphere, we must first be aware that we're not necessarily psychotic and broken when we fail to adjust behaviors to improve some facet of our lives.

Most of our relationship problems are not logical problems. They're emotional ones. So, high SAT scores and a PhD are going to be less valuable than developing our emotional awareness. EQ over IQ.

The emotions we feel are chemical. And chemistry is very powerful. I learned that in school while they weren't teaching me how to be a good life partner.

## THE WORST THING I'VE EVER DONE

The baby wouldn't come.

*Push.*

My wife was in pain. There was a growing audience of doctors and nurses. It must have been the most vulnerable she had ever felt.

I was twenty-nine. Clueless and helpless. Just standing there with my mouth half-open, I'd squeeze her hand and mutter "C'mon, baby," more to my wife than to the baby.

But, no baby. The labor had been a long one. Induced more than twenty-four hours earlier.

*Push.*

Our child was not coming. The doctors were monitoring heart rates and blood pressures and all the things we normally take for granted that can turn a typically happy occasion into a tragic one.

*"Okay. No more. We've got to take her to surgery,"* the doctor said.

I just stared, dumbly and wide-eyed. The doctor told me it would be okay. I wanted to believe her. A nurse handed me a pair of scrubs to wear.

Surrealism took hold as I was shuffled into the operating room where everyone there was preparing for emergency surgery.

My wife was exhausted. I'd never seen her like that. The anesthesiologist started doing his thing. Because I had never experienced anything like this, fear took over as I watched my wife's eyes roll into the back of her head—almost a total loss of consciousness.

I didn't know what was going on. Only that a bunch of strangers were cutting my wife open and that I didn't want her to die.

Everything was happening so fast. At 8:24 p.m., I heard crying.

*Holy shit. Our baby.*

A nurse carried a messy little bundle of human toward me.

*"Can you tell the sex?"* she said with a smile.

A boy. *I have a son.*

To my left, nurses were cleaning and poking and prodding a flailing, crying little boy whom I was now responsible for turning into a functional human being.

To my right, doctors were stitching up that baby's exhausted mother.

I looked left. *My son.* Then right. *My wife.*

They were going to be okay, everyone said.

Once he was cleaned and swaddled and outfitted with a teeny tiny baby hat, the nursing staff put our son in my arms. Mom had done every ounce of work—an understatement—and I got to hold him first. It seemed unfair. But exhausted and barely lucid, she just smiled at him. Mission accomplished.

*He was okay.*

*She was okay.*

My wife had just spent 158 years (in labor time) trying to deliver a baby and being cut open.

She was starving. The hospital gave her cold, shitty chicken fingers. I don't remember how much she ate.

Eventually, the baby was given to Mom. He needed to be fed.

Breastfeeding was not going well. Our stubborn little son wasn't cooperating. The brand-new mother must have been terrified and feeling so helpless.

It was late and I was getting tired. I had some people tell me that I should really try hard to get adequate sleep because between the two parents, it is helpful to have at least one of you mentally sharp for sound decision-making. I somehow got it in my head that I was going to go home for sleep and come back in the morning.

My wife was exhausted from the past two days and scared because *We have a newborn!* and the only people around to help were strangers.

She asked me to stay. She needed me to stay, she said, emotionally spent and crying.

"It's going to be okay," I said. "I can't help you, but the nurses can. I'll be back first thing in the morning."

My wife was as frightened and vulnerable and exhausted as she had ever been.

I understand now that she didn't want me there to "help," necessarily. She wanted me there because companionship and support provide people a sense of safety. There was a tiny little human who she was responsible for keeping alive and raising, and she believed that I was as invested in that process as she was. She wanted to know that someone had her back. That she was loved. That her son's father was reliable when life felt painful and scary.

But I thought she was acting needy and overly dramatic.

And on her very first night of motherhood—tired, crying, freshly stitched from surgery—I left her in that hospital room.

Alone and afraid.

O

I have what I perceive to be a sociopathic trait. I struggle with the ability to empathize with the physical pain of others.

When I read books, or hear someone describe something I've never seen, my brain dials up images, but what I visually imagine is almost never what reality ends up looking like when I finally get to see it. Maybe that's why I struggle with relating to the physical pain of others. Because I can't properly imagine it.

I am quite sensitive to emotional pain—especially if I have been through something similar to someone who is hurting or when I can adequately imagine what it would be like.

That matters for two reasons: I wasn't appreciating how much physical discomfort my wife was experiencing during pregnancy, and because I was an ignorant dipshit, I also failed to grasp the fear, stress, and anxiety she might have been feeling while worrying about both child delivery, first, then the following eighteen years or more of being responsible for the safety and well-being of an actual person.

I had been texting some of our closest friends from the chair next to her bed while my wife was in labor, updating them on her and the baby's status. I thought I had been doing something important.

She made it clear she wasn't pleased with that choice. She wanted me to be fully present and engaged, demonstrating my commitment to her, and reinforcing in her mind and heart that I would always be at her side through life's difficult moments.

*I would never consider something more important than the birth of my son.* But texting friends while my wife was in labor—no matter how uneventful or undramatic it seemed to me as it was happening—felt to her as if I valued doing what I wanted more than I valued her and the birth of our son in her most-vulnerable moments.

*I would never physically abandon my crying wife.* But that's what I did. She cried. She asked me to stay. But I left anyway because it was what I wanted to do.

I left my crying wife alone in a hospital room just hours removed from an emergency C-section, where she struggled to breastfeed a screaming child who didn't want to with nurses who made her feel like she just wasn't trying hard enough.

Why?

To sleep, shower, send photos to family and friends (smartphones weren't a thing yet), and revel in the amazing feeling of being a father to a newborn son.

I hope you believe me when I tell you how reasonable and justifiable it seemed at the time.

But in the context of my nine-year marriage, it's the worst thing I've ever done.

O

She wanted me there. The woman who would eventually leave. The wife whose eventual departure felt like uninvited heart-removal surgery. The deepest rejection and most intense pain I have ever known.

That same woman WANTED me there. Wanted to raise a little boy together. Wanted to be married for the rest of our lives.

But I shrugged her off. I had more important things to do just then.

"You're fine, babe," I said. "Everything's going to be okay."

The same thing the doctor had told me.

Turns out, we were both wrong.

# 4

# IS YOUR SPOUSE HURTING YOU ON PURPOSE?

I NEVER REALLY KNEW MY WIFE EVEN THOUGH WE WERE MARRIED for nine years and met when we were teenagers. Not because of any crazy spy shit or from deliberate attempts on her part to hide her identity from me.

I didn't really know my wife because for the entirety of our relationship I never invested the time, effort, and energy to really know and understand her. Some effort would have eliminated my blind spots and equipped me with the information I needed to avoid hurting her.

*"I'm so sorry! I didn't mean to! I had no idea this was such a big deal to you!"* That's the big defense in our relationships, right? I imagine this sounds familiar. In truth, it is the best-possible version of this "blind-spot" dynamic and yet it will still poison your relationships and end your marriage.

The more common version of this story involves one of us trying to convince our partner that they're overreacting—that whatever transpired SHOULDN'T be a big deal to them. That if they realize how insignificant the incident/comment/interaction/conversation was, or how silly the fight is, then they can stop feeling bad about it. *No one's upset anymore! Problem solved!*

That's what I did. I tried to make my wife feel better by explaining my feelings, believing I guess that she might adopt my version of events, thereby relieving her of the inconvenient pain, anger, or sadness she was feeling.

○

Something that frustrated me, and which frustrates many of the men and women I talk to in my coaching work, is the feeling that our partners are frequently "surprising" us with new complaints.

Right? Like, you're just going about your day, minding your own business, not doing anything that seems harmful to anyone, and—BAM—she's making her angry face and using her angry voice.

*Neat. Here we go again.*

Honestly, my wife would be hurt and/or upset by something she experienced, and my legitimate mental and physical reaction was to filter everything she was telling me through this idea of her being a petty, unfair, nagging, hypersensitive, overly emotional ingrate.

I thought SHE was the one making our marriage shitty. I seriously believed that.

When you think of yourself as a smart, kind, polite person who succeeds at work, has healthy social and professional relationships, and who always got along well with family members growing up, and the ONLY person who ever complains about you is your spouse (whom you promised to love forever, share everything with, and whom you perceive yourself to sacrifice most for), then it's easy to mathematically arrive at this conclusion because the sad and angry wife in this example is the statistical outlier. She's the one who is acting radically different than the rest of your interpersonal data sample. *Who am I going to believe? My own judgment plus EVERYONE I've ever known? Or this crazy woman trying to make me out to be the bad guy?*

So please don't interpret me as demonizing these defensive spouses or myself ten years ago. You can be legitimately decent and well-intentioned and still harm your spouse and marriage in your blind spots.

**Good people can be bad spouses. Good people unwittingly destroy their marriages.**

And one of the ways that happens is when spouses (in my experience, it's usually husbands) are "surprised" by their wives' expressed sadness or anger. Over and over and over again.

*How did this happen? How is it possible she's this upset about something I didn't see coming?*

The damage happens BECAUSE you didn't see it coming.

When you see children running in the house, or next to a swimming pool, or skateboarding in the middle of the street, the apparent dangers are obvious.

You see the potential hazards and can alertly work to avoid outcomes involving pain or injury. It's probably not because you're psychic. It's probably because you have the knowledge and wisdom that comes with experience and a nuanced understanding of these various situations.

The same things happen in our career pursuits and while engaged in our favorite hobbies.

Whatever we have spent the most time practicing, or reading about, or thinking about, or discussing are the things about which we have the most expertise. All of us have something.

I type fast and can usually string words together efficiently. I know a lot about NFL football, Marvel movies, bourbon whiskey, video games, the newspaper industry, cooking, poker, and chess relative to most people. For better or worse, I've invested a lot of time in each of those subjects.

I've also learned a lot about human relationships over the past several years because I've studied them, thought about them, written about them, and talked about them more than anything else.

Whatever we spend the most time doing and have learned the most about are the things in which we develop expertise or mastery.

Unfortunately, most of us never go to How to Be a Good Spouse University. We don't even attend How to Be a Good Spouse 101 in high school.

Many of us don't learn the things relationships require to function effectively until it's too late or dangerously close to the brink. It sometimes takes a serious shake-up in our comfortable lives before we are willing to start asking and answering the more difficult questions about who we are and why we do the things that we do.

○

I had a relationship coaching client in his seventies. Married thirty-six years. He was expressing frustration about hearing the same complaints from his wife for nearly forty years. (Feel free to laugh. I sort-of did even though it's probably more sad than it is funny.)

I asked him to grab a pen and paper and, in two columns, jot down the things that mattered most to his wife. One column of positive stuff. One column of negative stuff.

In other words, what are the things that affect your wife in good and bad ways? What are the things that move the needle for her emotionally in either direction?

My client couldn't name ONE thing. Not one.

"I don't really know, Matt," he said.

*Well. Gee whiz.*

"Respectfully, sir," I said, "you don't know your wife."

○

Imagine studying poker, playing in live games twice per week, playing online several times per week, and watching countless hours of it on TV.

I have poker textbooks that I would pore over. I would study the pros on television. I would analyze every nuanced decision the best players in the world were making. I would read recaps of tournaments or high-stakes hands in *Card Player* magazine for insight and inspiration.

And it worked. I got pretty good.

Now. Imagine being a woman who—in every decision she makes, large and small—factors her husband into the equation.

What to have for dinner. When to broach certain subjects with me. What plans to make for the upcoming weekend. What gifts to get my parents for the holidays or their birthdays—something that hadn't occurred to me before she mentioned it.

There were almost no decisions my wife would make throughout the course of a day that didn't take into account how those decisions would affect me or our son.

Compare that to me.

I woke up, maybe worked out, drove to work, did work stuff, drove home, and then maybe I'd cook or clean up the kitchen. Maybe I'd mow the lawn if it were getting embarrassing. One or two days per week, I'd vanish for poker night. When I was home, maybe I was playing online poker, watching a movie or TV show that I liked, or "managing" a fantasy football team.

You know? Minding my own business after a day where I went to work, cooked dinner and cleaned up the kitchen, and then sat down to watch, read, or play something. Harmless enough.

So, that's why I always thought it was bullshit when she'd be upset with me about something.

Because I *didn't do anything*.

And I was right. I didn't do anything. I was SURPRISED by my wife feeling upset or neglected or disrespected by something I either did or didn't do.

Imagine if I'd given the list of things that affected my wife both positively and negatively even half of the attention I gave to trying to master poker or win my fantasy football leagues.

Maybe if I had a nuanced understanding of the sorts of things that caused my wife to feel pain it would have occurred to me just how hurtful it must have been for her to see me put so much time, effort, and energy into mastering a card game she had no interest in, and which took me away from her and our home several hours per week, while never investing even a fraction of that same disciplined focus, effort, and energy in her. Or into our marriage. Or into optimizing our home life in a way that might have helped her feel seen, heard, respected, cherished, desired, and supported.

What if I had KNOWN my wife? What if I really had understood who she was? Her hopes and dreams. The very specific reasons that things I thought were petty created pain for her. What if I—with well-practiced expertise—had developed mastery-level skills for marriage and a comprehensive understanding of who she was and what mattered most to her?

Someone who knows their spouse with the same mastery they have of their profession or favorite hobbies is a person capable of anticipating his or her partner's emotional, mental, and physical needs in real time. Without surprises.

The "invisible" or unpredictable bad stuff doesn't happen because we can anticipate it. Imagine a life without being "surprised" with another "petty" complaint. Imagine a partner who never complains or criticizes because she or he is in a constant state of having their needs met. Of being considered. Of being validated. Of being respected. Of being loved.

I don't know what you're best at in life. But I'm pretty sure you were mostly pedestrian, if not bad, when you were just getting started and didn't even know what you didn't know.

Likewise, maybe you're accidentally shitty at various aspects of participating in your relationship. Maybe you're routinely confused by your partner's emotional reactions to things you do or don't do.

And just maybe, putting in the work of understanding and knowing things about them will mitigate much of the conflict and discomfort in your marriage.

Just maybe, when we are tuned in to our partners and develop expertise on the things that affect them—both good and bad—we are able to anticipate and meet their needs in real time. Without surprises. Because these potentially hurtful things are no longer happening in our blind spots.

We see the sharp corners. The boiling pan on the stove. And we become more mindful and cautious. No more *"I had no idea!"* No more *"I didn't mean to!"*

Maybe that's how we help prevent a lot of pain, and more effectively soothe it when it happens. Maybe that's how we turn frustrating, unhealthy, and disconnected relationships into ones everyone wants to take part in.

I didn't know my wife. But, if I'd chosen to, I could have. And that would have changed everything.

## THE ROAD TO HELL IS PAVED WITH GOOD INTENTIONS

Imagine being married to someone who looked at you every day and said, "Screw you and your feelings. I want you to suffer and I'm happy that you are feeling pain. I'm going to run off to my lair now and plot more ways to hurt you."

I don't get to decide what's right and wrong or good and bad, but I feel secure in encouraging anyone married to someone like that to run for the hills, stat.

While people are sometimes hurt by someone claiming to have good intentions, and while that hurt should be validated no matter what, I believe there's merit in knowing whether you're living with someone looking out for your best interests or someone secretly thinking up ways to make each day suck more for you.

I spent years defending myself against my wife's grievances by imploring her to grant me more patience and forgiveness on account of me loving her and having her best interests at heart.

And so instead of validating her pain and seeking to understand it more fully, I'd pivot the conversation to how unfairly she was treating me. It's because I was really bad at husband-ing.

But imagine if she KNEW that I wasn't hurting her intentionally? The way she knew her infant son wasn't trying to sabotage a peaceful night of sleep when he woke up crying.

Might that have helped? I like to believe so.

Millions of spouses and relationship partners who feel perpetually unseen and unheard by their partners might challenge this idea, but I can't stress enough how innocently intentioned I believe the Invalidation Triple Threat response pattern to be, where we tend to invalidate the thoughts and/or feelings of our partners or defend our actions anytime they result in hurting or upsetting the other person.

Remember, the Invalidation Triple Threat shows up the same three ways over and over again:

1. We contradict the intellectual experience our partners share.

2. We contradict the emotional experience our partners share.

3. We defend our character and justify our actions, based on what we knew at the time, and imply that we will repeat in the future this same behavior that our partners JUST finished trying to explain was in some way harmful.

I do not believe that husbands are thinking, *"My wife just said that Event X happened like a stupid idiot. She's just a woman with a small brain. A third the size of my superior man-brain. It's science."*

The problems we have in our romantic relationships and marriages are not the results of a bunch of bad people doing a bunch of bad things and trying to hurt one another on purpose. The problem is that there are a bunch of decent and well-intentioned people legitimately unaware that something they're doing or saying (or perhaps something they're not doing or saying) is hurting their partner.

We'll talk about self-care and healthy personal boundaries later, but let's get this idea out of the way right now: If you're married to or in a committed relationship with someone you believe to be INTENTIONALLY harming you, then I encourage you to reconsider being in that relationship. I am not aware of any healthy relationships in which one of its members is constantly plotting and executing new forms of misery on the other partner.

But if you are married to someone who loves you and who you very specifically chose to spend the rest of your life with because you believe them to be a good person, then please consider that moments of conflict and the pain of trust erosion are the result of accidentally inflicted wounds—NOT intentional abuse or neglect.

One of the greatest lessons from divorce and adulthood has been the realization that **unintentional pain and unintentional trust betrayals will end your relationship as surely as intentional ones will, only slower.**

○

One exercise I sometimes ask coaching clients to focus on is developing the skill of telling the story of a specific incident from their spouse's or romantic partner's perspective.

Novelists often write scenes involving multiple characters, and the only person whose beliefs, feelings, intentions, and motivations are understood are those of the protagonist. The main character or hero. We see the world through their eyes.

When we recount stories in which we were involved, we filter those stories through OUR beliefs, feelings, intentions, and motivations. You can see where I am going.

Here's an idea. There's a strong argument to be made for making ourselves a side character in these stories.

If you can articulate the way a moment felt to your partner and provide your understanding of the context for why they felt as they did while also providing details about how your own behavior could have positively or negatively influenced it or improve things moving forward, then you're someone your partner can trust.

Accidentally (*I didn't mean to!*) or ignorantly (*I didn't know!*) hurting someone STILL hurts them. And people don't trust things, situations, or people who hurt them, no matter how well intentioned everyone involved might be.

For my former client Donovan, a significant pain trigger for his wife turned out to be a pair of dehumidifiers near the family's basement laundry room.

The kind, loyal, but increasingly sad woman would make her way to the family's basement nearly every day in service of her family's laundry needs. She dutifully washed everyone's clothes—her own, her husband's, and her children's—in the washing machine, then transferred those clothes to the dryer, and afterward folded or hung up each item for everyone in the house.

And while she toiled silently doing this lonely, invisible, thankless work for more than two decades, she would sometimes glance over at the two dehumidifiers designed to prevent basement dampness and help protect their home from water damage. Their silence announced that they weren't running. Their lit-up red indicator lights communicated that the units' bins were full of water and needed to be emptied before they would start running again.

Those red lights communicated something else as well: *Your husband didn't take forty-five seconds to come downstairs and empty the water bins again even though you have kindly asked him dozens of times and he promised that he would.*

Maybe he was upstairs in his lounger having a beer and watching baseball on TV. And maybe she was downstairs folding his underwear.

Sometimes she would cry and feel like the loneliest, most invisible, most unimportant, most unloved person in the world. She strongly considered ending a marriage that had taken up most of her life—a marriage and family that her entire identity was wrapped up in.

And all the while, Donovan was upstairs in the family room watching the next pitch, oblivious to her growing, suffocating sadness.

Sometimes his wife would say something about the dehumidifiers being full and needing to be emptied. Sometimes she would talk about how disappointing and upsetting it was for her that the dehumidifiers were consistently full, leaving her with a choice—do it herself even though he had promised he would or go interrupt whatever he's doing to be a "nag." To be "the bad guy" even though that's never who she wanted to be.

And maybe sometimes when her sadness or frustration would boil over, she would tell Donovan how much this situation upset her. And I think he felt a lot like I did when my wife would communicate her disappointment and pain because of something I did or didn't do.

*Good grief. She's whining about the dehumidifiers again. Imagine what she'll do during the next power outage, or God forbid, a death in the family. She really needs to get a grip!*

Donovan's wife had a different perspective.

*I spend every moment of my day serving my husband and children, and he can't even prioritize giving up one minute of his evening or weekend to empty the dehumidifiers. Something I care about isn't worth him remembering. I don't matter enough to him.*

And then, silently, alone with nothing but her thankless laundry work to comfort her, she would cry.

Donovan is an awesome guy and a loving, involved father. He just had a blind spot about these dehumidifiers. Because he was never in the same room as part of his normal routine, he often forgot about them, and had never considered the emotional impact this situation was having on his wife.

Now, he is dutifully emptying the two dehumidifier containers every day. Not because he's submitting to the nagging wishes of his ungrateful wife but because he loves and respects her, and he truly appreciates how much she sacrifices so that he and his kids can have the life that they do.

He never even thought about how sad and lonely and afraid she used to feel while folding his clothes and noticing those two dehumidifier indicator lights. He didn't know what those lights meant to her. But now he does and he's doing something about it.

He has made the decision to not allow the woman he loves to feel pain because of his blind spots. He wasn't going to allow her to feel lonely and unloved simply because he was previously too busy and comfortable to remember the dehumidifiers. So now he does. Now, he embraces the opportunity for his wife to look over at those dehumidifiers and feel seen and respected and considered and safe and loved because the indicator lights are dark, and the two units are running.

Once he was able to connect dehumidifier indicator lights with very real emotional experiences his wife had been having, he learned how to connect other moments—and other conversations about those moments—with very real emotional experiences she was having.

He learned how to mindfully love his wife—not just with empty platitudes and brittle reassurances—but with love in action. The invisible became visible.

Emptying dehumidifiers equals building and maintaining trust with his wife. Donovan doesn't care about the dehumidifiers running nearly as much as she does. But he very much cares about her feeling hurt because he was too busy or too comfortable not paying attention.

Donovan did the work. And now she feels a new level of being loved and respected in their marriage.

I'm so proud of him and grateful that he is doing the work I was too big of a wimp to do in my marriage.

When we can explain how our partner feels, and how our own words and actions contributed—and WHY—and then have them nod their heads in agreement because we are accurately describing what they think and feel, we forge an environment of safety and trust in our relationships. When they recognize that we truly see them and know them and that they can count on us to anticipate their needs as we navigate life together, then we have truly earned their trust.

Those are the relationships capable of lasting a lifetime.

## EMPATHY IS THE #1 SKILL WE NEED TO SUCCEED IN RELATIONSHIPS

The most psychologically and emotionally impactful example of empathy I have ever encountered came from an unlikely source—a video game. And not only a video game but an apocalyptic video game rife with horrific zombie-ish creatures in varying stages of mutated undeadness, along with plenty of human-on-human violence among the few remaining people alive on earth.

The game is PlayStation's *The Last of Us Part II*, the 2020 sequel to the original *The Last of Us* from 2013, which prior to Part II, was probably the coolest game I'd ever played.

(**Note:** The following contains spoilers for the video games *The Last of Us* and *The Last of Us Part II*—and possibly for the live-action screenplay adaptation in the works at the time of this writing, so if you're interested in watching or playing this story as its creators intended, you should skip ahead to the next section. I have no interest in spoiling great stories.)

In the original *The Last of Us*, the protagonist is Joel, whom the game player controls—a man who tragically loses his young daughter in the chaos that was day one of the zombie apocalypse. The story quickly zips us a decade or two into the future, where an aged, hardened Joel reluctantly gets roped into escorting a young teenage girl, Ellie—the only known human to be immune from the mutated fungus that turns people into monsters—across a war-torn and creature-infested United States, narrowly escaping death more often than not.

On this journey, Joel grows fond of Ellie and they develop a father-daughter-like bond. The game even puts us in control of Ellie for a little while. As players, we in turn grow fond of both Joel and Ellie. We *care* about their survival. Near the end of the original story, playing as Joel, we learn that to make the serum doctors hope will save humanity, Ellie will have to die.

Joel is not okay with this. We, as Joel, slaughter dozens of people to save Ellie from certain death. After we dramatically and heroically save Ellie, the game ends as Joel and Ellie drive off toward some uncertain future.

Enter *The Last of Us Part II*.

Early in the game, Joel goes missing. Under the guise of needing help, a young woman we don't know lures Joel to a hideout where she and her friends have set up camp. We learn that they have spent years trying to hunt him down. They tie Joel up and beat him.

As Ellie, we immediately go out in search of our missing friend and father figure. We eventually locate the camp and sneak in before getting rushed and overpowered by a group of people. Ellie is pinned to the floor by strangers. She sees Joel across the room, tied up, beaten and bloody. She cries out for him.

The woman responsible for luring Joel back to the camp and beating him mercilessly—her name is Abby—is implored to "finish it" so the group of strangers can return to their home.

Abby grabs a golf club.

Ellie watches. Horrified. Helpless. Screaming. Pleading for Joel's life.

But Abby hardly hesitates. In the most brutal, breathtaking, ruthless act I've ever seen play out in a video game (which you'll recall are traditionally designed to be fun), Abby ends Joel's life with one sickening swing of the club in her hand.

One of the other guys walks up and spits on Joel, now dead. After spending hours *being* this man as the protagonist of this story, this entire scene guts you. Ellie is left, bloodied and sobbing on the floor as the gang of murderers departs.

End of scene.

Ellie, as Ellie does, goes on a revenge mission. And we happily play along. We must have vengeance for Joel.

Until, several hours into the game, something insane happens.

We suddenly find ourselves playing as Abby. Joel's killer.

And it's weird because she doesn't seem so evil. She's walking around her postapocalyptic colony, and everyone seems to think she's pretty great. She's kind to others. Jokes with friends. She has a tender moment with the community's pet dogs.

In a later flashback scene, we learn the uncomfortable truth about the final stanza in the original *The Last of Us* game. Abby's father, it turns out, had been the medical surgeon tasked with extracting from

Ellie whatever was needed to manufacture a vaccine that was supposed to save humanity.

We see Abby, as a young teenager, interacting sweetly with her father and playing in and around the hospital.

These were not evil doctors. Ellie was being brought to them voluntarily. And that's when Joel went on his violent rampage at the end of the first game to save Ellie's life, only now we're seeing it play out through the eyes of this young girl, Abby. As Abby, we see the carnage of Joel's heroism.

Dead security. Dead medical staff. And, most poignantly, a dead father.

As game players, we didn't hesitate nor did we feel any compunction about ending the lives of these people we assumed to be bad guys, but Neil Druckmann and his writing team at Naughty Dog turned everything upside down and inside out and forced us to consider our actions from the perspectives of others.

It forced us to watch a previously happy, young, innocent teenage girl experience the horror of finding her murdered father and bearing witness to the violent deaths of many innocent people.

And finally it hits you: *When you experience this story as Abby, Joel is the monster.*

I wasn't suddenly on board with her killing him with a golf club, but, in the context of the way this postapocalyptic vision of the world operates, I *understood*. What seemed heartless and cruel at the beginning of the game ended up being the moral equivalent of the revenge mission we had already been on with Ellie leading up to this moment, only now we have perspective and emotion from both sides.

Before the game ends, you must fight the heroine Ellie as Abby, and then later fight Abby as Ellie. And holy shit. All of it. Just, *holy shit.*

While the game cleaned up most of the major awards it was eligible for, it released to a bunch of controversy and internet hate from detractors. Some of that criticism was rooted in people's anger with the game's writers who killed off the original protagonist. The original hero.

It is my experience that the best stories ever told involve painful loss. And this one is no different. Without the high-stakes loss, maybe we wouldn't be invested enough to care about what Abby's motivations were for the killing.

The power of perspective shift can't be overstated, and it's so important for us to do that within our relationships (and probably with everyone).

○

Empathy is a skill, one we need to effectively navigate our human relationships. But in order to practice empathy, we must first make a choice, a choice that, in my experience, many people (particularly men) seem unwilling to make. To successfully empathize with others, **we must make the courageous choice to be vulnerable.**

It's so easy to feel lost when we don't have a tangible sense of purpose and meaning in our lives. The human connections we make by being vulnerable with others (those incredible *I see them, and they see me* moments) help to provide that sense of purpose. Remember how divorced men die more often than married men? In many cases, these guys feel simply that they have less to live for in the absence of partnership, which, ironically, dissipated in many cases because of their refusal to demonstrate vulnerability with their spouse.

If we're unwilling to be vulnerable, then we're unwilling to share the whole truth about who we are. Without sharing the whole truth about who we are, we can never be as trustworthy as relationships require to remain healthy.

"Vulnerability isn't good or bad. It's not what we call a dark emotion, nor is it always a light, positive experience. Vulnerability is the core of all emotions and feelings. To feel is to be vulnerable. To believe vulnerability is weakness is to believe that feeling is weakness. To foreclose on our emotional life out of a fear that the costs will be too high is to walk away from the very thing that gives purpose and meaning to living," wrote Brené Brown in *Daring Greatly*. Brown is the world's leading researcher on vulnerability and shame and the world's thought leader on empathy. "Vulnerability is the birthplace of love, belonging, joy, courage, empathy, and creativity. It is the source of hope, empathy, accountability, and authenticity. If we want greater clarity in our purpose or deeper and more meaningful spiritual lives, vulnerability is the path."

## MISDIAGNOSING MY DIVORCE

I'm an idiot, but I'm like a smart-ish idiot. I've always been fairly analytical, curious, and interested in getting to the WHY behind anything that interests me. I want to know how or why something happened and how or why someone or something behaves as it does.

My mental aptitude is in the top 10–15 percent of the general population if you place any stock in standardized academic testing.

And even though I'm kind of smart-ish, when I applied all of my brainpower to figuring out the WHY behind my wife wanting to divorce me when our marriage was coming apart at the seams, I settled on an incorrect conclusion. (That conclusion being that she was mistaken regarding my intentions. Combined with her propensity for letting her silly girl feelings cloud her judgment, my wife was quitting. Breaking her promise. Being unfair. I believed all of that.)

Misdiagnosing a health condition is bad. We can't treat or fix what we don't recognize or understand. Making missteps in a root-cause analysis following a disaster will in no way serve our efforts to prevent that disaster from happening again.

Similarly, if we misunderstand what went wrong at the end of a relationship, then we are likely doomed to repeat the experience.

When we misdiagnose problems during the relationship, then we spend our time and energy on things that won't actually make anything better. This is why people sometimes feel as if they're working hard on their relationship only to continue being fed shit sandwiches from their seemingly ungrateful partners who aren't responding emotionally the way the misdiagnoser wants them to.

That was me. A misdiagnoser.

My wife's father—my father-in-law, a man I loved and respected—died out of nowhere one autumn day. We'd all had dinner together the night before. Everything was fine. Happy. Fun. The very next night, I learned the tragic news from a phone call and was suddenly facing the task of telling my wife the most painful news she would ever hear.

The following month was a blur. I tried to play the role of good husband and good son-in-law for my wife and extended family.

But that woman wasn't my wife anymore. She seemed like someone else, and it seemed as if she saw me as someone else. Someone she couldn't or wouldn't allow to get too close to her.

I thought it would get better eventually. It never did. I lost my wife when her father died.

So, what did I do? I pointed to that tragic life event, interpreting it as my wife mishandling the situation emotionally. I convinced myself that my "overly emotional" wife was putting her feelings ahead of more important things like our marriage and family.

Here's the worst part in terms of the modern-day divorce crisis: I'd argue that that story makes sense. It's easy to believe.

Many thoughtful, intelligent people might agree with that initial analysis, make a snap judgment about my ex-wife or me, and never put any energy into digging for more truth.

"Yeah, Matt. That's terrible. Something similar happened to my other buddy, Trey," one of my friends might have said. "She's being selfish, and putting her sadness ahead of your marriage, and now your family is suffering for it. Sorry, man."

It doesn't always matter what's true. It doesn't always matter what's real. People will act on their beliefs—independent of whether we agree with those beliefs or even realize that person has them.

If you value your relationship with someone, it will be helpful to come to terms with this truth. When we love people, we must honor THEIR experiences—THEIR reality—to connect with them on an emotionally healthy level. More on that in a bit.

## THERE'S FAMOUS PRECEDENT FOR SMART PEOPLE CONVINCING THEMSELVES OF BULLSHIT

For 1,500 years, early astronomers used Ptolemy's geocentric model of the solar system to create astronomical charts. "Geocentric" refers to Earth being the center of the universe with everything in the sky orbiting around it.

Today, we know this isn't true. Around the year 1510, mathematician Nicolaus Copernicus became suspicious and theorized that we were actually the ones moving around the sun—which came to be known as the heliocentric model and is credited for starting the Scientific Revolution in the sixteenth century. Later, Italian genius Galileo Galilei proved the heliocentric model of the solar system that most of us understand today.

But for 1,500 years prior, every educated person in the world believed the sun revolved around Earth. And it wasn't because everyone was a bunch of stupid morons. Given the mathematical parameters and limited technology of that time, you can prove—legitimately—Ptolemy's model, a fact that delighted me as a fifteen-year-old high school student in astronomy class.

For 1,500 years, the smartest people in the world—every scientist, navigator, educator, and thought leader—knew how the sun, moon, and stars would move in the sky. They could "prove" it convincingly by accurately predicting what would happen next in the sky, even though everything about their prediction model was based on limited and incorrect information.

People can believe things that can't be proven—big and small. Please don't get hung up on the countless religious and political examples of this in world history but do consider that there are people in your personal life who might believe something about you or about your relationship that isn't true, whether or not you realize it.

And if you're constantly operating outside of THEIR reality, you're bound to disagree with them, fight with them, confuse them, frustrate them, anger them, and hurt them.

Oh yeah—this is how your marriage ends.

○

Most people are familiar with the Bible story of David and Goliath. It's frequently used to characterize any underdog scenario in life where an individual or competitive sports team might be facing seemingly insurmountable odds.

With apologies to Old Testament writer Samuel, I'm going to share three verses from the famous David and Goliath story, but I'm going to replace one word three times, because doing so might save your marriage, and I'm pretty sure Samuel would want that.

> 48 As the Philistine moved closer to attack him, David ran quickly toward the battle line to meet him. 49 Reaching into his bag and taking out a cotton ball, he slung it and struck the Philistine on the forehead. The cotton ball sank into his forehead, and he fell facedown on the ground.

> 50 So David triumphed over the Philistine with a sling and a cotton ball; without a sword in his hand he struck down the Philistine and killed him.

Holy shit! Did you just see that, guys?

Little shepherd David just smoked that giant Hagrid-looking sonofabitch right in the forehead with a small piece of balled-up cotton fibers and dropped him like third-period French class!

Wait.

That's a bunch of crap, right? Bollocks? Stupid? Impossible?

You guys ever see a movie or read a book where the story's protagonist knows something really important and tries to warn everyone about it but no one believes her or him until something horrible happens later and everyone goes, "*Ohhh. Holy shit. Voldemort REALLY is back from the dead, terrorists REALLY have taken control of Nakatomi Plaza, Freddy Krueger REALLY is murdering teens in their dreams, genetically modified dinosaurs REALLY are a threat to kill amusement park guests on Isla Nublar, future murder bots called Terminators REALLY are travelling through time to try and kill various members of the Connor family! I should have believed them! Now I feel like a huge dick!*"?

This is what our spouses experience when they attempt to communicate that something is wrong and we treat them like they're assholes for saying so. They're the people desperately trying to communicate important truths, but we're all "Berpa-derpa-derp! Relax, Francis. Have a drink! Everything's fine!"

We're being the huge dicks who don't believe the people who need us to. Because everything is NOT fine.

Sometimes, we see a cotton ball hurtling through the air and bouncing softly off someone else—our spouse perhaps—which is then followed by them freaking out as if that harmless cotton ball actually hurt them.

*What a bunch of drama-queen psychos.*

We get so focused on their whiny bullshit over that cotton ball hitting them that what they're actually saying hardly registers with us. And what they're actually saying is that, for them, it WASN'T a cotton ball hitting them. It was a stone. And it really fucking hurt. And now we're treating them like they're weak or delusional for feeling the very real, tangible pain that they know they are feeling.

We are concerned with their ability to process information within the framework of reality, right? How scary is it to live with a person who literally can't tell the difference between what's real and what's not?

When someone feels as if they're being hit with stones, how many

THIS IS HOW YOUR MARRIAGE ENDS 111

times do you imagine they'll stick around, despite our passionate pro-
tests that they're seeing and feeling things that aren't really there?

## WE MUST CHALLENGE OUR OWN ASSUMPTIONS, AND CONSTANTLY REMIND OURSELVES WHERE WE ARE AND WHAT WE'RE DOING

I have to keep reminding myself, every day. It's difficult. Not because
it requires some Herculean mental or emotional effort but because it's
just so damn easy to get caught up in the busyness and white noise of
the All The Time and "forget" that other people often see, hear, and
feel life happening around them much differently than we do.

And when we operate on our default setting, that's when we're most
likely to experience conflict with others, not because we're all looking
for a fight but because we're all perpetually busy trusting our own judgment and perceptions about every little thing that occurs.

We often speak and behave from a place of certainty, routinely
resulting in us being assholes whom others don't enjoy being around—
especially our romantic partners since they understandably hold us
to higher behavioral standards.

People often use logic and reason primarily in the service of supporting their preexisting beliefs rather than exploring and considering new
ideas that might challenge them or make them uncomfortable. The bot-
tom line is that, as people, we can feel as if we KNOW something even
when we actually don't.

It turns out that we make a lot of decisions, even something arbi-
trary like whether to go out with friends or stay in and watch TV, based
on our MEMORIES of some emotion we might have felt years ago.

And it turns out that our memories are totally shit. Psychologist Dr. Elizabeth Loftus, a heralded memory researcher, and the person who taught the rest of us that eyewitness testimony can't be considered a smoking gun in courtroom criminal trials, can prove it.

"One of the things that I and other people who do similar work have shown is that once you have an experience and you record it in memory, it doesn't just stick there in some pristine form, you know, waiting to be played back like a recording device," Loftus said in a podcast interview recorded at the 2018 American Psychological Association convention. "But rather, new information, new ideas, new thoughts, suggestive information, misinformation can enter people's conscious awareness and cause a contamination, a distortion, an alteration in memory . . ."

We routinely misremember past events because our brains unconsciously apply present-day emotions to events that happened years ago. Basically, we just make shit up as we go along.

*"But Matt! Doesn't that call into question every damn story you or I have ever shared about anything, ever?!"*

It DOES. Scary, huh?

One of the things that can help is to constantly remind yourself that you're a fallible human with a faulty brain that is shedding more and more brain cells every day. To choose to be a little less certain, every day, all of the time.

Zen masters in Eastern philosophy call this "beginner's mind," and it's an idea championed in Tom Vanderbilt's book *Beginners*, in which he warns of a psychological condition known as the Dunning-Kruger Effect, which "famously showed that on various cognitive tests the people who did the worst were also the ones who most 'grossly overestimated' their actual performance. They were 'unskilled and unaware of it.'"

This condition manifests most often when we evolve naturally from a total newbie to someone who, as the saying goes, "knows just enough to be dangerous."

Vanderbilt notes that doctors "learning a new spinal surgery technique committed the most errors not on the first or second try but on the *fifteenth*" and that airplane pilot errors don't peak in the earliest stages of gaining experience but most often when they have accrued about eight hundred hours of flight time.

People also experience this when visiting a strange place for the first time. We tend to soak up every foreign sight, sound, taste, custom, and landmark when we're first experiencing it, but after a few days in the same place, we naturally become more familiar and comfortable with our surroundings, and as a consequence, we literally notice less than we did before. This is why Vanderbilt has a habit of always taking the most notes on his first day in a new place: because he understands that is when he's most likely to notice the rich details.

This phenomenon speaks to the white-noise blind spots in our personal lives. How we're capable of walking by small piles of clutter in our homes or how we can eventually stop obsessing over some minor defect we discover on our vehicle's paint job or how we can wake up next to an especially attractive, desirable, loving, wonderful, worthy human being every day for several years and "forget" to notice how blessed we are.

## HOW DO YOU FEEL IN 65 DEGREES FAHRENHEIT?

My friend Lesli Doares, a couples therapist and podcast host, reminded me during a conversation that we can objectively know that the air temperature is 65 degrees, and have everyone agree that it is, because we can check ten different thermometers, all of which will confirm it.

Then she reminded me that people get into trouble when discussing whether 65 degrees is warm or cold, comfortable or uncomfortable.

I often use this 65-degree thought exercise as a framework for thinking about how we can more effectively consider our partner's experiences when we make decisions.

For example, let's pretend we generally feel comfortable in 65 degrees but know that our partner feels cold in the same air temperature.

This is about acknowledging your partner's experience in 65 degrees with thoughtful action rather than invalidating it with a sales pitch about how she or he is wrong to feel uncomfortable since it's an obviously comfortable temperature given your individual feelings about it.

Can we adjust the temperature if we're indoors? Or if not, could we choose to go somewhere warmer than 65 degrees on our partner's behalf?

If we must or agree to go somewhere that's 65 degrees, how might we consider our partner's experience beforehand?

Could we communicate ahead of time that it will be 65 degrees when we get there so that they can factor it into their clothing choices? Can we acknowledge that we are aware that it's a temperature that's uncomfortable for them and that it matters to us? Could we offer any support or assistance to help them be more comfortable in 65 degrees?

Might we mindfully grab a sweatshirt or jacket for them? An extra blanket? Might we thoughtfully sit near a heat source or somewhere out of the wind?

These are the unspoken actions that communicate "you are loved" and that I fear our partners too often fail to experience, leaving them to wonder whether we actually know them, or even care to.

○

We are so good at being stuck inside of our own heads and bodies. We are so good at defaulting to all of our beliefs and opinions being "normal" or "good" or "correct," and we are often blind to how things we never considered impact others because those same conditions don't impact us or cause us any pain or discomfort.

This happens all of the time, every day, in our beliefs and conversations that extend well beyond our romantic relationships. But that's a conversation for another time.

Do you ever make quick, thoughtless decisions that your spouse or relationship partner indicates is an inconvenience or pain point for them?

Like me, are you quick to dismiss them because you "know" just how unimportant those minor inconveniences truly are?

And if so, is it possible that these "little things" aren't the actual problem in your relationship? Could it be that what our loved ones actually crave is to be considered in our decision-making? To be worthy, in our minds and hearts, of always being important enough to include in our calculations—no matter how deceptively minor or inconsequential we might believe these calculations to be?

○

Pain sucks.

Some people enjoy the muscle burn after a hard workout because it feels like progress. Others like the achy remnants of vigorous bedroom activities, or headaches the morning after a fun party, as a reminder of the good time.

But we can mostly agree that pain in most forms and at most times is a predominantly negative experience. Hurt someone long enough or hard enough and they won't even be the same person afterward. It's a big deal.

My go-to defense when my wife was upset with me in our marriage was to say I didn't do it on purpose. To me, it felt unfair for her to be mad about whatever the thing was or AS mad as she sometimes was.

Inflicting damage intentionally is a universally frowned-upon thing. When your actions result in harm to other people or their property, the penalties in every criminal justice system I know about are most severe when the damage was intentional.

Accidents are sometimes punishable as well but usually with softer penalties. They're often labeled "negligent" or "reckless."

Whenever my wife was mad and I thought she was charging me with murder when my crime was actually driving too fast in a construction zone, I'd get defensive and pivot the conversation to her lack of justice instead of her expressed pain.

My marriage fights mostly consisted of me invalidating my wife's complaints under the premise that I considered them petty or unworthy. I treated her arguments as illogical. And because, in my mind, her arguments lacked logic and reason, I categorized them as wrong.

I was right. She was wrong. And since I believed that, she was the real rabble-rouser in the marriage and nothing was ever my fault.

I was either accidentally a master manipulator or an intolerably oblivious moron. Because both my ex-wife and I are socially competent, we didn't have many disagreements in front of others. I don't remember ever being pulled aside so someone could point out any of my douchebaggery. That's probably because their relationship arguments looked and sounded exactly the same.

I was months into divorce before the truth found me:

- This is what most marriages and relationships look like. Most couples have the same, predictable fights and outcomes.

- *Holy shit. I WAS hurting her in a very real way.* (We all get outraged when people physically strike others, but emotional neglect is less perceptible to everyone except for the person experiencing it, and it's hard to feel outraged by something you don't realize is happening.)

- I never knew that my actions were literally causing pain because I didn't believe her when she told me. *Did I think she was lying?* No. *I guess I simply thought she was wrong.*

- The intense pain from divorce was my first real taste of emotional pain. I'm not talking about how we feel when the girl at school doesn't like us back, or even when our parents get divorced when we're little. I'm talking about BREAKING on the inside.

- That experience gave me the ability—for the first time in my life—to consciously empathize with others.

○

When two sober, healthy, and seemingly functional adults love one another and promise to do so forever, it seems reasonable to expect that to work more than half the time.

But it doesn't. Half the time it's Hindenburg dot com. (Read: crashes and burns.)

Most people are born; grow up without the information they need to have healthy, functioning relationships; get married with a bunch of people patting them on the back and congratulating them; bring children into their flimsy world; and then even though most people are well intentioned and trying their best, it often breaks and turns to shit.

Why? Because we were unaware. We just—didn't know better.

When we're in it—fighting with our spouses and feeling betrayed because they don't seem to be loving us as they promised to on our wedding day—we sometimes feel like they're deliberately causing us harm. And that hurts more than the thing they're doing. That feeling that they would WANT to hurt us. That's what hurts the most.

## HOW TO KNOW WHETHER YOUR SPOUSE IS HURTING YOU ON PURPOSE

You ask them.

Don't roll your eyes. This is important. Ask them. Effectively. We rarely ask ourselves or others the right questions.

*What are the right questions?*

**The right questions challenge our assumptions and beliefs and force us to consider an alternative.**

A better way.

Author Matthew E. May shared this story about the advent of the Polaroid camera, which predated digital technology and was the first camera to offer near-instant access to whatever photo we just took:

*"Back in the 1940s, Edwin Land was on vacation with his 3-year-old daughter. He snapped a photograph of her, using a standard camera. But she wanted to see the results right away, not understanding that the film must be sent off for processing.*

*"She asked, 'Why do we have to wait for the picture?' After hearing his daughter's why question, Land wondered, what if you could develop film inside the camera? Then he spent a long time figuring out how—in effect, how to bring the darkroom into the camera.*

*"That one why question inspired Land to develop the Polaroid instant camera. It's a classic Why / What if / How story. But it all started with a child's naive question—a great reminder of the power of fundamental questions."*

○

What question should we ask?

*"Do you know why I am upset with you?"*

Or.

*"When you think back to [insert personal experience] and how that hurt you—do you understand that I feel similarly right now?"*

Or a more cooperative exercise.

*"In an effort to try to understand you and not fight about this, I want to try to make your argument for you. I want to say what I believe you think and feel, and why you think and feel that way so that you know I understand you. I was hoping you would agree to do the same for me. Will you?"*

**Until your partner demonstrates beyond doubt that they can articulate accurately your point of view, you can safely conclude that THEY DON'T KNOW HOW YOU REALLY FEEL.**

The significance of that can't be overstated.

I don't think any of us sensitive to the other side of divorce could sleep at night if we had a true picture of the numbers of broken homes, broken families, broken people, broken children, broken spirits that have resulted from this one little notion . . . two people didn't really know how the other felt.

What if all the pain and dysfunction is just one big misunderstanding?

## WHEN PAIN OR DAMAGE OCCURS, DO INTENTIONS MATTER?

Most of my coaching clients will remember me noting that we can obey every conceivable traffic law and perform every known best practice for safe driving but still hit someone's beloved family pet with our vehicle because there was no way to see it before it darted into traffic.

We can be remorseful and accept responsibility for our role in the loss of a family's pet without having intentionally caused harm and without accepting blame.

Intentionally killing a family's dog strikes me as a more heinous act than accidentally doing so. I believe most would agree. But there's a cold math calculation to deal with all the same: People lost a member of their family. There will be sadness and grief.

We have a choice to make as to how we want to show up in that moment. We can make it about us, and prioritize defending our character and emphasizing our blamelessness, or we can make it about them—sympathizing, empathizing, and apologizing for their loss, despite having done nothing wrong.

Do intentions matter?

You get to decide. I'm no divorce advocate, but I also won't hesitate to encourage people to end relationships with people who would intentionally harm them. There's no path to a healthy, loving, sustainable relationship with an intentional abuser.

There aren't many people who struggle to understand how little kids or their parents might cry and hurt upon learning of their pet being killed in an accident. It's as obvious to most of us as how a large man might be felled by a stone striking him in the forehead with enough force.

But there are scores of people who struggle to understand how someone might feel hurt because of a dish left by the sink. To them, that seems as illogical and absurd as a large man being killed from being struck by a cotton ball.

Everyone has a different list of things that can hurt them. Our pains are not universal, just as our level of comfort in 65-degree air is going to vary from person to person.

When we don't know our spouses—when we're not experts about who they are, what harms them, and what brings them pleasure or joy—then we are a constant threat to hurt them regardless of how much love we feel for them and regardless of our intentions.

The alternative is to get intentional about NOT hurting people. It's a choice we get to make every day.

*If any of us want to succeed in dating, marriage, parenting, or friendship, we need to replace this habit of judgment with something else. Curiosity. Empathy. Encouragement.*

# 5

# WORDS DON'T ALWAYS MEAN WHAT WE THINK THEY MEAN

"THERE ARE THESE TWO YOUNG FISH SWIMMING ALONG, AND they happen to meet an older fish swimming the other way who nods at them and says, 'Morning, boys, how's the water?' And the two young fish swim on for a bit, and then eventually one of them looks over at the other and says, 'What the hell is water?'"

This is the opening parable that the late novelist David Foster Wallace shared while giving a commencement speech to Kenyon College graduates in 2005, just a few short years before he died by suicide. The speech is called *This Is Water*, and I try to listen to it every couple of months or so because it reminds me of who I want to be and how I want to show up in the world.

"Suicide is such a powerful end, it reaches back and scrambles the beginning. It has an event gravity: Eventually, every memory and impression gets tugged in its direction," writes David Lipsky in his book *Although Of Course You End Up Becoming Yourself*, which documents his five-day road trip interview with Wallace at the tail end of Wallace's 1996 book tour for the novel *Infinite Jest*.

In Wallace's *This Is Water* speech, he spends a minute on the subject of suicide, and I feel something gutting every time I hear him talk about it, knowing now what his audience didn't know then.

*Event gravity.*

Wallace was the most awake—the most *alive*—person I have ever encountered. Wallace—through his work—taught me how to flip a switch and pay attention. *To really pay attention.*

Because it's the opposite—an absence of awakeness; this white-noisy, comfortably numb, routine-filled life many of us find ourselves in, hopping back and forth between busily doing life stuff and pleasurable distraction—that prevents us from seeing how our actions or inaction cause pain in others.

Of course, you're under no obligation to give a shit about this pain happening to other people in your blind spots. I'm not here to judge you. I'm just here to say that my obliviousness to the ways in which things I said and did hurt others—namely, my wife—is the condition most responsible for the implosion of my personal life. And as a relationship coach, this lack of awareness is one of the primary pain points I see impacting relationships in all stages.

Blindness. A blissfully (until it wasn't) ignorant, thoughtlessly selfish, perpetual lack of awareness.

And if the quality of your marriage or other close relationships is something you value, then I'd invite you to spend more time considering how the things that happen while you're busy not paying attention are what will slowly damage, and eventually destroy, your most precious relationships.

Not paying attention is a habit. A dangerously comfortable one.

In Wallace's speech, he says the most important thing I've ever heard regarding the human experience:

"The really important kind of freedom involves attention and awareness and discipline and being able truly to care about other people and to sacrifice for them over and over in myriad petty, unsexy ways every day," Wallace said. "That is real freedom. That is being educated and understanding how to think. The alternative is unconsciousness, the default setting, the rat race, the constant gnawing sense of having had, and lost, some infinite thing."

I rarely think about Wallace without the staggering punch of his suicide popping into my head. That knowledge permeates my experiences with his writing or writings about him.

Because suicide has an event gravity.

Divorce has its own kind of event gravity. Divorce is a life ended. A story ended at worst, a page turned at best.

And what's interesting to me about divorce is how *regular* a bad marriage looks and sounds.

Like many of us, my wife and I had the audacity to discuss other people's marriages in our car rides together after parties or other social gatherings in which other couples' humanity might have been on display. It's in our nature to compare others' lives to our own, but it is often another sign of a lack of awareness.

"They won't be married in ten years, but we will be, babe," I probably said. And she probably knew better.

A marriage destined to fail and one that will last fifty-plus years will look and sound the same to other couples at the party or dinner table.

Often there's no spectacle, no loud, obvious drama that communicates to everyone in earshot that these two don't have a prayer of making it. Because, to most of us, the conversations between the two people who won't stay married sound pretty much like the conversations every other couple is having.

It's just two people talking. *What could be so bad about that?*

Divorce has event gravity.

Too many of us don't see divorce (or the end of a major relationship) coming until we're choking on its inevitability. Until we find ourselves fighting for our next breath, wondering whether life is ever going to feel like life again.

○

Two common occurrences are responsible for destroying trust in our relationships:

1.  An event or situation in which one or both partners feel hurt by the other, and

2.  The conversation we have about that hurtful event or situation.

The event is one thing, but the conversation is usually where shit hits the fan. And after that happens enough times, people often want to divorce because of how badly they hurt.

And if that sounds maddeningly unfair to you, we are in total agreement.

I'm repeating myself because I have to think about new ideas over and over and practice new behaviors like my response patterns many times before new habits are formed. If I'm not mindful of my default-setting beliefs, then I'm prone to think and speak from a place of certainty. And since we're people, and we're mistaken more than we'd all like to be, blind certainty can get us into trouble.

As has been shared, I always thought that I was a good person. Smart enough to know right from wrong and to discern bullshit from truth as well as being nice enough to know the difference between mistreating someone and not.

So, when my wife would characterize something I had said or done as "mean" or "bad," my brain would sometimes take in those words and ideas, let them roll around for a beat or two, and conclude that my wife was wrong about me.

All of this was happening in nanoseconds. My brain was all *What the?! She's girl-spazzing again! It's probably that time of the month!* And my body was like *Grrrrrrrr. I'm really mad. Fight or flight?*

This will sound familiar to all of you. For me, sometimes I chose Flight. I would attempt to disengage and walk away, confused, feeling defeated, and not wanting to hear the person I loved the most hurl what I perceived to be unfair or false accusations at me.

Sometimes I chose Fight. At my worst, I'd respond emotionally, insisting that she was actually the one in the wrong here because I was neither doing nor being whatever she seemed to think I was. At my best, I'd calmly attempt to share my alternative perspective, believing that she was mistaken or misinformed, and that once I explained my side, she would recognize the mix-up as clearly as I did.

Day after day, coaching people in relationships on the brink, I hear the same things. Constantly and most of the time unconsciously, we invalidate the lived experiences of the people we love. With great conviction, we tell them to their faces that their thoughts and beliefs are wrong. We tell them that their feelings are wrong. And we tell them that their treatment of us is wrong—that it's unfair.

Not because we're trying to be awful or cause harm (although that line gets crossed in the heat of many arguments). It's because this is what we really think and feel. And so, despite everyone's best intentions, one of us trusts the other just a little bit less than we did the day before.

A ticking clock too quiet to hear. A countdown that seems too inconsequential to address.

## YOUR RESPONSE PATTERNS ARE HABITS YOU CAN CHANGE

People don't fall into the trappings of the Invalidation Triple Threat because they're "bad people" or because they're "dumb and wrong." They fall into this marriage-ending Same Fight cycle because they're good people. Because they're smart.

When my wife told me that I was doing a bad thing or feeling a bad thing toward her, I KNEW she was wrong. I didn't think she was wrong. I knew she was.

When you spend your entire life literally avoiding hurting others as much as possible every step of the way, it sounds like lunacy when your spouse is suggesting that you're out to get them.

You'll recall that the Invalidation Triple Threat repeatedly shows up in the same three ways:

1.  We contradict the intellectual experience our partners share.

2.  We contradict the emotional experience our partners share.

3.  We defend our character and justify our actions, based on what we knew at the time, and imply that we will repeat in the future this same behavior that our partners JUST finished trying to explain was in some way harmful.

This is—in my estimation—a totally normal and expected response to someone who is saying something to you that you believe to be either mistaken or fundamentally unfair.

It makes sense for you to try to set the record straight or to correct what feels like a wildly off-base character attack.

It's impulse. This isn't something we deliberate on. If someone says something our brains calculate to be wrong or unfair, the easiest and most obvious thing in the world is to respond accordingly.

Habit. Autopilot. Our default settings.

This is how your marriage ends. This is how. In your everyday conversations.

○

If I continue to hyperfocus on my wife's incorrectness (*But I'm totally right about this!*) or on how unfair she's being (*How can she say and feel this stuff about me? I would never, ever do anything to try to hurt her!*), then I'm going to spend the rest of my marriage impulsively and reactively responding to my wife in ways that invalidate her experiences.

And this can't be said or thought about enough times—invalidation erodes trust. Always.

And once trust has eroded to the point of no longer being present in a relationship, then the relationship will cease to feel safe.

And when safety and trust are absent, there are only three possible endings:

- Shitty relationship until it ends.

- Shitty relationship that lasts a lifetime.

- The restoration of safety and trust and a marriage that both participants want to be a part of.

○

If we don't hold on to this principle—that trust MUST be present to maintain a healthy relationship, keeping it at the forefront of our thoughts and maintaining awareness of it by shining a light on it instead of comfortably allowing it to recede back into the shadows of our blind spots—then we are a constant threat to hurt people we love without realizing it.

We will slowly sabotage our relationships by habitually operating on default settings, saying and feeling whatever feels natural—*without considering how our words and actions affect others.*

This is the magic of David Foster Wallace's *This Is Water.* This reminder to pay more attention to what we think about.

*"If your total freedom of choice regarding what to think about seems too obvious to waste time discussing, I'd ask you to think about fish and water, and to bracket for just a few minutes your skepticism about the value of the totally obvious,"* Wallace says.

We struggle to notice ever-present things, things that are All The Time.

Whirring fans, chirping birds, or the sounds of city traffic. The indicator light on my stovetop is designed to warn me that a burner is still turned on. It broke somehow and never shuts off. I don't notice anymore. Guests often do.

If we were fish who had spent every moment of our lives in water, would we even know what water was?

The No. 1 skill that we need to succeed in our most critical human relationships is empathy. But it can be difficult to practice when we struggle to instinctively relate to what others might be going through. We automatically empathize with people dealing with something we've also lived through. It's easier to demonstrate compassion for people with whom we share similar experiences.

In the case of my marriage, I think I was pretty decent at showing up as loving and supportive whenever I agreed with my wife. If she tried to communicate an idea or feeling or experiences that made sense to me, I was rock-solid at politely expressing my understanding and, if called for, my compassion for what she was feeling.

The problem arises for all of us when we don't agree or can't default naturally to an empathetic position. When pain or sadness or anger or anxiety is expressed by someone we love and their reaction doesn't make sense to us or elicit the same emotional response, we too often invalidate their lived experience.

If my wife's thoughts didn't pass my personal *Is she right about this?* test, then I responded honestly, which thoroughly invalidated her thoughts and beliefs.

If my wife's feelings didn't pass my personal *Are her feelings appropriate for this situation?* test, then I responded honestly, which completely invalidated her emotional experiences.

On autopilot, as a matter of habit, I told my wife that her thoughts and feelings were wrong or crazy EVERY TIME they didn't align with my own thoughts and feelings.

Empathy—to see the world through someone else's lens—is a relational skill not all of us are taught during our formative years. We either figure it out or continue to hurt the people we love. Let's figure it out.

## FORMING BETTER HABITS BEGINS WITH IMPROVED SELF-AWARENESS

Habits are the compound interest of self-improvement, says *Atomic Habits* author James Clear. If you want better results, then forget about setting goals. Focus on your system instead.

This applies as much to your mental and behavioral habits within your romantic relationships as it does to your eating and exercise habits.

The most effective way to change your habits, Clear says, is to focus not on what you want to achieve but on who you wish to become.

"Your identity emerges out of your habits," Clear writes in *Atomic Habits*. "Every action you take is a vote for the type of person you wish to become. No single instance will transform your beliefs, but as the votes build up, so does the evidence of your new identity. This is one reason why meaningful change does not require radical change. Small habits can make a meaningful difference by providing evidence of a new identity. And if a change is meaningful, it is actually big. That's the paradox of making small improvements."

The quality of our relationships will be determined less by major events and more by the accumulation of thousands of little things that— any one of them—by themselves might seem completely innocuous.

As author and speaker Simon Sinek says, you can go to the gym, work out, come home, look in the mirror, and see that nothing has changed. You can even go to the gym the following day for another difficult workout, come home, look in the mirror, and once again feel the disappointment of nothing changing.

One might conclude afterward that going to the gym and working out doesn't improve our appearance or health if that's the way we choose to measure it. But what Sinek encourages business leaders to consider is how to think about measuring results differently. And I'm asking you to consider applying these same ideas to your intimate relationships.

If you fundamentally believe working out is the right course of action, and follow it, you'll eventually get in shape, he said.

"It's not about intensity, it's about consistency," Sinek said in an interview with entrepreneur Tom Bilyeu. "[If you only] go to the dentist twice a year, your teeth will fall out. You have to brush your teeth every day for two minutes. What does brushing your teeth twice a day for two minutes do? Nothing. Unless you do it every day twice a day for two minutes."

When we become mindful of how our habits affect trust and intimacy and the overall quality of our relationships, then consistent behavior and consistent decision-making within the "thousand little things" of everyday life becomes what will help our relationships thrive, or if we make different choices, slowly result in their decay.

If you continue to live in your experience only and insist that your thoughts and feelings are superior or more correct than your partner's, responding as you always have, then you will continue to inadvertently invalidate them and erode trust between the two of you. Moment by moment the bond that connects you is being eaten away. And sooner or later it will snap—at a time we won't necessarily see coming.

o

I didn't know how to notice my own thoughts. Either that, or I was stuck in a habit of not bothering to try.

We end the toxic, relationship-ending habit of invalidating our loved ones' experiences only after realizing that's what we're doing.

You can't replace the habit if you don't notice it in the first place and then decide that you want to.

There's something appalling—nearly unforgivable—about the things we forget, like, 98-ish percent of our existence. For example, we forget that we breathe. We breathe more than 23,000 times per day on average. There's literally nothing we have done more times in life than taken a breath. Yet, we hardly notice our breathing.

We forget that we are not promised tomorrow. Today may be our last. This conversation may be the last one we ever get to have with someone. Virtually all of us would say and do things differently if we knew this interaction would be our final one.

We forget many of the opportunities we have to be grateful. Health. Money. Shelter. Clothing. Transportation. Family. Friends. Employment. Education. Abilities.

There's always something to be deeply thankful for—something we're taking for granted. Our health and closest loved ones seem to be the most obvious victims of our unintentional neglect.

My blindness to the All The Time is why my marriage ended. I think it's why most marriages end.

There are many ways to frame and slice the conversation about how love dies. But, in my case, underneath all of the specifics is a simple and difficult truth: *I didn't remember to actively love my spouse.*

Like, you could say I forgot. I feel shitty about it, and I'd feel even worse if I didn't know that pretty much everyone suffers from this in some form or fashion.

We grow numb to the things we feel All The Time.

We grow deaf to the things we hear All The Time.

We grow blind to the things we see All The Time.

I hope it's clear that I felt love for my wife. The same way I feel grateful for breathable air.

I just forgot somehow to actively demonstrate it in the way that would have saved everyone involved a lot of pain and suffering through the years. Sometimes, when you have a near-death experience with a Jolly Rancher, you remember how neat it is to be able to breathe without out a delicious piece of hard candy lodged in your windpipe.

*"News at 11, a local man was found dead in his parked vehicle this afternoon. Law enforcement officials at the scene declined to com-*

*ment on the active investigation, but we were told off the record that there's no evidence of foul play, and that a bag of Jolly Ranchers candy was found on the passenger seat, suggesting the man likely died from a choking incident as you might expect from a small child. None of the man's co-workers admitted to being friends with him. Reporting live from Cleveland, Ohio, this is Johnny McJohnson. Back to you in the studio."*

I had a serious problem with forgetting to actively love my son. He's amazing. And he's been my entire world since his mom and I stopped living together.

And even though that's true, and even though I've never known love like the love I feel for him, I have gotten really upset with him before (almost always when getting ready for school, where his priorities sometimes seemed to be anything except stuff that would help us accomplish our goal of getting to school on time with as little stress as possible).

And I could get pretty mad when I wasn't being my best self. Because I know what he's capable of, and I know how smart he is, it sometimes felt almost as if he were intentionally sabotaging my efforts to get us where we needed to be. (*I know. The irony isn't lost on me. I promise.*)

And sometimes, he and I would exchange words and attitude, and maybe this was all happening on a school morning where I wouldn't be picking him up later that day, per his mother's and my shared-parenting arrangement. Maybe it would be two or three days before I would see him again.

So, sad and angry dad drops off sad and angry son only to have both of us feel crappy about it for a while. Both of us would have chosen to go back in time and do it differently if we could.

And since he was in grade school and I'm supposed to be the adult, I needed to take action. Because doing the same thing over and over again more or less guarantees the same results over and over again.

*I could make myself a sign*, I thought. *I could get a tattoo. I could set reminders on my phone. I could write it on my calendar.*

I could have done a lot of things. But ultimately, I chose a simple black flexible wristband. One of those rubbery ones like the #LiveStrong bands that former cyclist Lance Armstrong used to pimp before he admitted to doping and a bunch of people stopped thinking he was cool.

I bought a box of them. They all have cliché motivational words on them that annoy me, but in this case, the word "Focus" is apropos. I now wear a mostly nondescript, small, black rubber wristband on my left wrist. There is nothing special or noteworthy about it. Unless I'm wearing short sleeves, no one would ever know it's there.

My Focus wristband has one job. Only one job. To remind me to actively demonstrate intentional love and patience toward my favorite person in the world. He is my life's greatest gift. And it's pathetic that I get angry with him and speak to him in ways his young mind might interpret as me saying he's not good enough or that might communicate to him that I'm not immensely proud of him.

Jolly Rancher jokes aside, what if on one of those mornings, I never made it to my destination? What if the last thing he remembered about me was me being angry with him at school drop-off, only to never have the chance to speak again or remind him that there is NOTHING he could ever do or say and no amount of frustration he could ever make me feel that would equate to my love for him lessening somehow?

Nothing about that seemed okay. So, I ordered a pack of these silly wristbands. And, you know what? It works.

My Focus wristband reminds me to smile and laugh at him clowning around when he's supposed to be brushing his teeth. My Focus wristband reminds me that a few lost minutes here and there are not even in the same universe as important to me as him knowing his father loves him and feels immense pride in him.

My Focus wristband literally triggers intentional patience, resulting in a 90 percent reduction in anything resembling an emotional outburst and a much more mindful father not carelessly "forgetting" how much he loves his son.

I know it might seem silly, this small thing. This wristband with only one job.

I was skeptical as to how effective it would be. I shouldn't have been.

**When we MINDFULLY, INTENTIONALLY invest our mental and emotional energy in those we love, it sticks. Because we know what's at stake.**

Someone somewhere doesn't know how much you care about them. They don't have any idea how much they are loved and cherished. What super-tiny, subtle shift can we make to keep our minds attuned to what matters most to us and help us maintain discipline, better communicate our love for others, and walk the walk in our daily lives?

What small thing can we do today to invest in and protect our life's most-sacred relationships?

I paid about $15 for a pack of wristbands I only needed one of. But can you guess how much it's worth? There's not enough room here to write out the number.

O

This idea of mindfulness is a near-constant topic of conversation with my relationship coaching clients. Of paying attention. Because the alternative is to default to the same habits that have eroded trust in our past relationships and current ones. The alternative is to allow the people we love the most to honestly question whether they are actually loved.

In the context of habits, the way I've come to think about this is that I needed to learn how to notice my thoughts. I had to learn how to observe what happens when someone says something with which I disagree or perhaps a criticism or accusation that somehow makes me uncomfortable.

And one day it occurred to me that I was JUDGING my wife when she would share her pains with me, often triggering an Invalidation Triple Threat response from me. I was always evaluating what she was saying or doing or feeling, measuring it against what I believed to be "right" or "appropriate" or "fair" or "the best way."

When I judged my wife's thoughts—her opinion or interpretation about something that happened—to be "correct," I was loving and supportive.

When I judged her thoughts to be Less Than somehow, I contradicted her. *Invalidation.* I didn't mean it this way, but my wife must have heard "*No, you dumb, silly person! Your brain isn't working correctly! Here's the smart-person way to think about this.*"

When I judged my wife's feelings about a particular situation to be appropriate (meaning her feelings aligned with how mine would be in a similar scenario) then I was empathetic and supportive.

But, whenever I judged her feelings to be faulty—an overreaction or some hypersensitive reaction—I would try to convince her that there was a better, healthier, more appropriate way to FEEL about the situation. Feelings just like mine. "*Bless your little feelingsy heart, babe! You're just being a weak little crazy girl right now, but there's hope because I'm here to explain how you're SUPPOSED to feel! One day, with practice, you'll be a smarter, more-fair person, and then these things that upset you will no longer upset you!"*

I didn't notice this process of judging my wife's thoughts and feelings while we were still married. It occurred to me only after I was through judging her for giving up on us.

To have any chance at participating effectively in future relationships, I knew I had to break this habit—this routine, thoughtless, near-constant invalidation dance that couples do almost every day, slowly paper-cutting themselves toward a bleed-out that will end their relationship.

○

Again, I'm not saying I know what's right and wrong and you should always do things a certain way. I don't believe it's morally reprehensible to disagree with someone, which they may experience as invalidation. I don't think it's "evil," or even "bad."

What I do think is that it erodes trust. Every time. And after enough trust erosion, marriage breaks. Any meaningful relationship will break.

And if you, as I do, value the concept of NOT behaving in ways known to damage other people and our most precious relationships, then I think there's merit in deciding we're no longer going to allow the people we love or our relationships to suffer because of things we have the ability to influence.

Coaching clients sometimes ask me what they're supposed to do when they disagree with their spouse. "What am I supposed to do? Just agree with everything she says for the rest of my life and not have any thoughts or opinions of my own?"

No.

But that's exactly the way I used to think about it. I thought it was so unfair that anytime I didn't agree with my wife, I was the bad guy. *Holy shit, am I not allowed to think and feel differently about this than you?*

I was confusing validation and agreement. They're not the same.

I am both allowed to disagree and capable of disagreeing with someone while still validating their very real experience with whatever we're discussing.

I am capable of being unfazed personally by a spot or two of toothpaste in the bathroom sink while understanding that my wife might feel much differently about it and then discussing the cleanliness of the bathroom sink on her terms—not mine.

"Empathy is a strange and powerful thing. There is no script. There is no right way or wrong way to do it," wrote Brené Brown in her bestseller *Daring Greatly.* "It's simply listening, holding space, withholding judgment, emotionally connecting, and communicating that incredibly healing message of 'You're not alone.'"

I needed to learn how to care that whomever I'm speaking with is suffering in some way and how to respond to them in a way they would experience as understanding and supportive. I needed to learn how to care about that rather than running the situation through my personal litmus tests. *SHOULD this person feel that way? SHOULD they believe this? Isn't that weak or silly or unhealthy or wrong?*

This is my worst habit as a human being when I'm operating on my default setting. This insta-judgment I might make about another person's beliefs or feelings and then minimize or dismiss them when they don't align with MY beliefs or emotions, with absolutely no awareness as to how intolerably arrogant this makes me.

If any of us want to succeed in dating, marriage, parenting, or friendship, we need to replace this habit of judgment with something else. Curiosity. Empathy. Encouragement. **Anything but judgment.** Anything but measuring other people's subjective experiences against our own.

"The real reason habits matter is not because they can get you better results (although they can do that), but because they can change your beliefs about yourself," James Clear says.

## THE MONSTER UNDER THE BED THEORY

Imagine getting a phone call. You answer. A stranger on the other end of the line identifies him- or herself as a law enforcement agent.

You feel a little flutter of anxiety.

The law enforcement official names someone you love dearly. Maybe it's the name of a family member.

*"There's been an accident. I'm so sorry. Would you be willing to come downtown to identify the body?"*

Shock. Disbelief. Disorientation.

Maybe the most unspeakably painful feeling that you didn't know your mind and body could experience without dying.

You end the call.

Maybe everything's in slow motion. Surreal. Or maybe you rush into action because you're the kind of person who functions well in emergencies, even when you're falling apart on the inside.

Minutes go by. Maybe hours.

Maybe you text or call others to share the tragic news.

*I can't believe they're gone.*

You arrive at the morgue. They take you to a back room where you'll identify the body for the coroner or medical examiner. You're a mental and emotional wreck.

They pull back the sheet. You stare down at the face and motionless body of someone you can't imagine living without, your worst fears realized.

And then this person jumps off the table: "*SURPRISE! You can't get rid of me that easily!*" and all of the morgue workers and cops laugh and laugh and laugh and point at you while you try to process what just happened.

It doesn't matter that someone you loved dearly hadn't really died and had pulled the sickest, most-savage prank imaginable. Your brain and body experienced the situation as if you'd actually lost someone precious to you.

Your mental and emotional reactions were consistent with the tragedy having actually happened. What's real, it turns out, doesn't always align neatly with painful feelings of fear, sadness, or anger.

Sometimes, caring about someone is much less about what we perceive as real or valid and much more about understanding just how bad someone else might be feeling and then demonstrating concern for the pain they feel even if we don't feel it ourselves.

## "DAD, I'M SCARED. THERE'S A MONSTER UNDER MY BED."

The thought exercise I lean on most to help me habitually respond to other people in the ways I perceive to be healthy and trust-building is to imagine a child crying because they are afraid of a monster hiding under their bed.

A monster you and I know isn't there.

I like the extremeness of not just having a difference of opinion on the matter. This is a subjective experience in which facts are clearly on our side as adults who have, often over several decades, ruled out the possibility of magical creatures lurking under beds or hiding in bedroom closets.

We *know*. My son believes something that isn't true. He's afraid of something that isn't real. And it's really tempting to leverage this "correctness" as a methodology for dealing with the situation.

And so, we've arrived at the moment—the moment in which we're going to choose how to speak and act toward someone we love who is feeling terrible emotions (fear and anxiety).

I have a choice to make.

And it's tempting for me to, annoyed and impatiently, tell this little boy how silly and foolish he is being—crying and afraid because of something I understand to be a figment of his imagination.

"Listen, bud. There's no monster under your bed. Monsters aren't real. There's literally nothing to be afraid of, so please don't act like a baby. You're too big to cry over make-believe stuff. I don't have time to deal with this right now. I'm trying to watch the game. It's time to toughen up and be my big boy. Please go to sleep. Everything's fine."

I could say something like that. And I wouldn't be "wrong." I wouldn't be "bad." I wouldn't be hurting this child purposefully.

This is where the work of choosing comes in. The work of being aware. Of being "awake."

Who do I want to be in this moment? Do I want to be "right"? Is that the most important thing to measure? When I was still married, I used to think so. I believed that "being right" was important and worth fighting for. That getting emotional based on things I believed to be untrue or unworthy of feeling bad about was the wrong thing to do.

What happens after I, in all of my superior adult wisdom, leave that bedroom?

My son is still afraid. My assurances that his fears were based on something that isn't actually dangerous did not alleviate him of his fear and anxiety. He's still afraid.

Only now, maybe he's crying. Alone and in the dark. And he just learned something about his father.

*"If Dad doesn't think the scary thing is scary, then he doesn't care about how I feel. If I feel bad about something that Dad doesn't think is important, he's not going to do anything to help. Telling Dad about the things I'm afraid of doesn't actually make anything better. It only makes me feel worse."*

And there lies my son in this totally fabricated—but plausible— scenario. Sad. Afraid. Abandoned. Hurt.

He just learned that he can't trust his father when he's afraid of something. And now, maybe he's going to grow up keeping all of his fears to himself. Maybe now he'll go through his teenage years hiding his personal battles from his parents because trying to include them in the past did nothing to help. In fact, doing so only causes more pain.

What is the value in being "right" about this monster-under-the-bed thing? How did me knowing it was bullshit and trying to share that knowledge and "wisdom" with my son do ANYTHING to make a positive difference in either of our lives?

I've learned to value something more than the idea of "being right." And that's the quality of my relationship with the people I love.

Screw being right. It's bullshit. I mean, knock yourself out if winning these little knowledge battles with others gives your life meaning and completeness, but once I saw this toxic pattern I seemed forever stuck in, I committed to trying to abandon this habit of wanting to be right.

Because it's a choice.

You know what matters more to me than being right about whether a monster is hiding under a bed? My relationship with my son. That matters a whole hell of a lot more.

I want my son to trust me when he's afraid. When he's sad. When he's angry. When he feels bad. I want him to know his parents are people who are always going to show up for him and support him no matter how scary things might seem.

My little boy is crying in his room. Afraid of a monster I know isn't there. I have a choice. And the choice I've decided I want to make is to be the kind of person who prioritizes my loved ones' feeling safe and trusting me instead of trying to sell them on how right I am about their beliefs or feelings.

I submit that a more effective and healthy way to respond to a child who is afraid—who is experiencing very real, actual fear, independent of how little we understand why, and regardless of how irrational we think it might be—is to sit or kneel down next to them. To hug them.

"Hey. I am so sorry that you feel afraid right now. You know, I've been afraid before too. Many times. It feels really bad to be scared.

"I'm here. I wish I could take your fear away, but I don't know how. I only know how to promise you that you're not alone. I love you so much, and no matter what, I never want you to feel alone. When bad things happen to you, they happen to me too. Okay?

"I'm pretty sure there are no monsters hiding under your bed. If it's okay with you, I'm going to turn on the lights and check for you, and when you feel ready, we can both look together if you want. Then, if you're confident that the coast is clear and that we don't have any monsters sneaking around here, maybe you'll feel good enough and safe enough to fall asleep."

I've decided that I want to be a person who values safety and trust in relationships more than being the "most correct" about stuff. I think that being the kind of person who mindfully chooses words and actions that promote safety and trust yields results that enrich our lives infinitely more than how many insignificant disagreements we "win."

○

It doesn't matter that when your seemingly sadistic family member or friend played the morgue prank on you, they weren't actually dead. You believed that they died, and while you believed it, your entire world was crumbling.

It doesn't matter how insane it seems to an adult that a child might believe there's a monster under their bed. That child is still feeling exactly how it would feel if there WERE a scary monster under their bed.

It doesn't matter how confused you are about why your spouse or romantic partner might feel as they do nor does it matter how irrational you consider their reasons to be. That person you promised to love and cherish is feeling actual pain. Actual sadness. Actual anger. Actual fear.

You don't HAVE to do the super-thoughtful parent thing and comfort the child who is afraid of the monster under their bed as described previously in order to be a person who loves their children.

It's not a right-or-wrong thing. It's not a good-or-bad thing.

I would argue simply that one way is an effective strategy for fostering an environment of safety and trust in a relationship built to be healthy and last a lifetime and that the less-compassionate, more-dickish *"There's nothing to cry about! Stop being a baby!"* version is more likely to produce strained, unhealthy relationships in the future.

We get to choose. And I want to be a person who chooses to comfort and support the people I love when they feel hurt or sad or afraid rather than try to convince them that they SHOULDN'T feel these things.

I believe that choice has profound implications for the quality of our relationships. And it's up to me to have the awareness and discipline to choose to show up in that way, even when I believe someone else might be mistaken or that they are feeling emotions that don't quite make sense to me as they're happening.

You don't HAVE to do the super-thoughtful and loving spouse thing when your partner communicates to you a pain or fear they're experiencing. I don't think about it as being right or wrong or good or bad.

I would argue simply that one way is an effective strategy for nurturing a healthy and loving and mutually beneficial relationship built to last a lifetime.

The alternative?

Strained, unhealthy, feel-bad, conflict-heavy relationships that won't last.

Love is a choice.

We can choose to be the kind of people who close the bedroom doors and tell our kids to shut up and stop being wimpy and afraid.

Or we can be the kind of people who sit down and listen. Who seek to understand. Who choose to care about things simply because the people we love care about them.

We can't prevent all injury. We can't prevent others from feeling sad or afraid.

But we can make sure that when they're hurt or sad or afraid, they know they're not alone.

# IT'S NOT A BROKEN CHARACTER DEFECT THAT NEEDS TO BE FIXED—IT'S A HABIT THAT NEEDS TO BE MODIFIED

I don't know how to fix some toxic, piece-of-shit human flaw inside of me that causes me to treat people in ways that will destroy my relationship with them. That might cause my wife to want to leave me. That might cause my son to pull away and keep me at emotional arm's length because he doesn't trust me to participate in his personal growing-pains battles.

I'm lost if I think about this stuff as a character defect. I'm at the mercy of whatever higher power you believe in or a lifetime of being victim to blind luck and everyone else's stupid beliefs and nonsensical feelings.

But when I think about my behavior—and others' behavior—not as some genetic fatal flaw I'm stuck with but as a habit I can practice changing to something positive and healthy, I find my sense of direction. A North Star.

Over and over and over again, I choose to be someone who mindfully speaks and acts in a manner that builds trust and promotes feelings of comfort and safety with the people I love. My relationships with these people are what I value most in this earthly life.

On my default setting, I remain a threat to judge and subsequently disagree with people and vocalize my opposition in ways that invalidate their experiences. I might gauge their beliefs to be wrong. I might consider their feelings to be inappropriate given the situation.

Maybe sometimes, I let them know in ways that inadvertently chip away at whatever amount of trust exists between us.

But with those I love and value most. With my son. With a romantic partner. With family and friends, I want to be someone who doesn't lazily fall prey to the toxicity of always trying to be right.

That scoreboard has no bearing on whether life feels good. In fact, the act of trying to score those points has consistently proven to make it worse.

It's not other people's responsibility to conform to my personal belief system and emotional calibration. It's MY responsibility to validate and empathize with anyone whose trust I crave and whose life I want to be a part of.

And to practice this habit of choosing the quality of my relationships over my inclination to dispute thoughts and feelings with which I disagree, I need only to have my mind's switch turned on to the Awake position. I need only to remember to remember.

And that's where David Foster Wallace's *This Is Water* serves as my foundational thought anchor for being the kind of human I want to be. The kind of person who doesn't inadvertently hurt people he loves and accidentally sabotage his relationships.

With that, let's have Wallace take us home:

*"I know that this stuff probably doesn't sound fun and breezy or grandly inspirational the way a commencement speech is supposed to sound. What it is, as far as I can see, is the capital-T Truth, with a whole lot of rhetorical niceties stripped away. You are, of course, free to think of it whatever you wish. But please don't just dismiss it as just some finger-wagging Dr. Laura sermon. None of this stuff is really about morality or religion or dogma or big fancy questions of life after death.*

*"The capital-T Truth is about life BEFORE death.*

*"It is about the real value of a real education, which has almost*

nothing to do with knowledge, and everything to do with simple awareness; awareness of what is so real and essential, so hidden in plain
sight all around us, all the time, that we have to keep reminding ourselves over and over:

"This is water.

"This is water.

"It is unimaginably hard to do this, to stay conscious and alive in
the adult world day in and day out. Which means yet another grand
cliché turns out to be true: your education really IS the job of a lifetime. And it commences: now."

## 6

# MOVE THE DOTS CLOSER: KEY RELATIONSHIP SKILLS TO PRACTICE AND MASTER

I WOULD JUST STAND IN THE KITCHEN, SHAKING. CONFUSED. Powerless. Fighting, and failing, to be understood. Defeated.

Rage. And nowhere to send it.

*How can the most beautiful thing I've ever seen make me feel most ugly? How can the person I give the most to be the person that makes me feel most worthless?*

Never in my life before, nor since, have I felt so weak or angry. I could never get over the idea that the person I loved most, for whom I felt as if I'd sacrificed most, and with whom I shared the most could be the person treating me the most unfairly.

And this is one of the most important realizations I've ever had: So long as I process everything my wife is doing and saying through the filter of MY thoughts and MY feelings, then I'm always going to have reason to defend myself. If I measure everything that happens through my individual lens of self—as if I'm the protagonist in the story—then anytime I am uncomfortable or feel mistreated or misunderstood, I will give myself license to try to set the record straight. To fight for MY wants and needs. To try to convince the other person that their thoughts and feelings are wrong.

And—*boom*—the Invalidation Triple Threat rears its ugly head once again. I never really had a chance to restore or maintain trust with my wife because I NEVER set aside my own thoughts and feelings to try to experience the moment as she was. I never considered HER as the protagonist in the story. I never wondered *What if I'm the villain here? What if it's me who is actually standing in her way? What if I am the one who is being unfair and inflicting pain?*

The truth is, I never even considered that idea. And in the moment that I was in, I was so pissed that I'm not sure I gave a shit about her feelings. I was too busy feeling like the victim of a hyperemotional, hypercritical tyrant. I was too busy trying to protect myself and defend myself against more unfair attacks and criticisms.

Talking about safety and trust earlier, I mentioned how I always wanted to be the person sleeping closest to the bedroom door. How I wanted to be with her in dimly lit parking lots. Et cetera. I believed I was someone who prioritized her safety.

And yet we would find ourselves in another fight in the kitchen, where she feels hurt—for the millionth time—and all she's trying to do is get me to understand and acknowledge her hurt. And instead, nearly 100 percent of the time, I would choose MY thoughts and MY feelings over hers. I wasn't thinking about her safety at all. Only mine.

I bet she felt rage just like I did. With nowhere to send it just like I did. Until the day came when she decided she didn't want to feel that anymore and made a different choice about where to live and about who she was going to allow to walk through the rest of adulthood with her.

And now, here we are. Strangers.

I took no responsibility for my own thoughts, feelings, and behavior in my relationship. If someone did something that resulted in me feeling bad, I blamed them for doing something wrong. And I did that, unironically, while almost never allowing someone else to feel bad because of something I did or said.

My marriage consisted of a bunch of things just happening to me. I never accepted responsibility for educating myself about emotional intelligence, about the importance of mindful empathy, or about skills I could have developed to be a better husband and co-parent.

It never occurred to me that being "a good person" wasn't the only prerequisite necessary to succeed in marriage. Successful relationships are comprised of two people who have and exhibit competent relationship skills, which I sorely lacked in my marriage. Skills I developed by thinking about, talking about, and writing about my divorce and human relationships, in general, until that work manifested into me being someone others wanted to talk to about developing their own relationship skills.

Had I understood and practiced these skills and thought exercises in my marriage, it would have helped—not only to prevent divorce but to foster an environment at home that would have allowed my marriage and family to thrive.

## RELATIONSHIP SKILL #1: CHOOSING SAFETY AND TRUST OVER BEING "RIGHT"

We have talked about this and it is clearly easier said than done. This skill takes practice. Like any habit you have ever developed or overcome. I know and you know that your aim is not to hurt your spouse. But please consider that your spouse is being hurt as a result of things you do or don't do, say or don't say regardless of your intentions. Anytime you choose to prioritize your beliefs and your feelings over your spouse's, they are going to feel just a little bit more hurt and lose just a little bit more trust in you and the relationship.

Nine times out of ten, this is the priority action item to emerge from the sessions with my coaching clients. When we operate on our default setting, and our spouses say or do things we calculate in real time to be incorrect or unfair, then we are going to respond accordingly, which will result in invalidation and contribute to further mistrust and disconnection.

If you have a habit of invalidating your partner whenever they try to communicate that something hurts or is wrong, this habit will eventually end your relationship.

As we have discussed, there's nothing wrong with trying to set the record straight or defending ourselves from unfair attacks. Absolutely nothing. BUT. When doing so also invalidates the mental and emotional experience of your romantic partner, you end up "doing nothing wrong" but still abandoning your spouse's mental and emotional needs in favor of your own. (Just as there's nothing "wrong" with telling a scared and crying child that there's no monster under their bed and to toughen up and go back to sleep. It's not "bad." It's simply harmful to your relationship with them because it compromises trust and, by extension, safety.)

Even when we are "doing nothing wrong," we are still capable of saying and doing things that erode trust in our relationship, and our relationship cannot last without trust.

Painful events aren't the only things that erode relationship trust. Relationship trust might be eroded furthest in the conversations we have ABOUT the painful events.

This is not about having some character defect that causes us to relentlessly harm our partner. This is about having a habit of reacting defensively whenever we disagree with something our partner (or anyone with whom we desire a healthy relationship) says or does.

We can choose to not do that. We can choose a better way. We can choose to intellectually process what our spouse says or does—disagree with it or feel confused by it—and instead of judging it as "wrong," we can simply choose curiosity to better understand it.

We can mindfully choose to foster an environment of safety and trust by validating, supporting, and comforting, rather than trying to discredit or argue, because **we choose to value the quality of our relationship with someone over winning a battle of ideas or feelings with them.**

Your response patterns are habits. When your partner says something you disagree with intellectually, or if they report feeling an emotion that you calculate to be unfair or inappropriate somehow, that is you JUDGING, or evaluating the merits of their thoughts and feelings. You're deciding whether another person's mental and emotional experiences are valid, and I hope you'll consider the inherent disrespect and self-absorption involved in that—determining that everything we think and feel is superior and more important than others' thoughts and feelings.

When I operate on my default setting, I will always express my disagreement or disapproval of someone else's thoughts and feelings if I calculate them to be wrong somehow.

So, I have to make the choice—the mindful, deliberate choice—that instead of judging someone else's experience to be wrong and trying to convince them of my mental and emotional superiority, I will try to understand all of the ways in which it makes perfect sense for them to feel as they do.

o

I like to imagine two friends back in the 1700s—before the field of optometry discovered the condition of color blindness. And I like to imagine these guys standing together, looking at a bushel of vegetables, or a field of flowers, and having a debate about the colors they see. One of them is color-blind and one of them is not.

And I like to imagine just how off the rails this conversation could go if neither person realized it was scientifically possible for two people to look at the same thing but see radically different colors. How many times does your asshole friend have to call the green thing "orange" before you lose it and accuse him of intentionally annoying you or, at minimum, of being a totally crazy person?

These two guys could end up at each other's throats.

"*Say it's green, dumbass! Say it NOW!*"

And of course, the other guy's like, "*The vegetable is orange, you stupid knob!*"

And it makes so much sense to me that two people who lacked maturity and self-control like me could get so pissed off over their idiot friend either being this intentionally dumb or this much of a psycho.

And then I like to imagine The Optometry Fairy magically showing up like Oz's Glinda the Good Witch of the North and being like, *"Hey! Chill out, dipshits! Neither of you are wrong. Neither of you are being dicks to the other. Neither of you are crazy. Here, try these on."*

The Optometry Fairy whips out some super-neato and futuristic color-blind simulating glasses and hands them to each guy. Suddenly, the guy with color-correct vision can see what his friend was seeing as his color-blind friend could of him.

*Holy shit,* they both think. *He wasn't wrong. He wasn't crazy. He wasn't trying to be an asshole. He—quite literally—saw something differently than I did. I didn't even know that was possible.*

I like to imagine the profound psychological and emotional impact this moment would have on these two friends. Just maybe, as I hope to do in my relationships, and as I wish for you as well, these two could spend the rest of their lives not emotionally jumping to the conclusion that the other person is automatically "wrong" or "bad" or trying to upset each other simply because they report seeing or feeling something differently than the other person.

I can be confused and frustrated by someone else's thoughts and feelings, and I can judge them to be wrong and say so, even though it will slowly erode our trust in one another until we have a shitty, toxic relationship. That's one option.

Or I can use it as a learning opportunity for myself. I can care that someone who matters to me is experiencing something they perceive to be bad or painful or terrifying, and I can choose to express some empathy and remorse that they feel bad somehow, and then I can do the work of learning WHY a particular event or a particular statement triggered the negative emotion.

I may never feel just as my partner does in a particular situation—just as I may never wake up in the middle of the night afraid of a monster hiding under my bed—but I can make the choice to love them, comfort them, validate them, support them, and seek to understand them.

I can always choose the quality of the relationship over my individual thoughts and feelings. And doing so is the difference between having relationships with trust and emotional intimacy and relationships without.

## RELATIONSHIP SKILL #2: KNOW YOUR PARTNER ALMOST AS WELL AS YOU KNOW YOURSELF

There are many ways to think about knowing—truly KNOWING—our spouse or romantic partner. I believe the first and most obvious way is to simply know our partner as well as the things we know the most about.

People study law and medicine. Others are automotive or aviation mechanics. And others still are restaurant line cooks or nail technicians at beauty salons.

Grocery store managers and corporate accountants know their work and workplaces on nuanced levels that I can't imagine unless I was exposed to them long enough and committed to learning what they know.

In addition to careers and vocations, people also demonstrate mastery in other areas of life. Aficionados. Cigars. Luxury handbags. Travel. Comic books. Sports betting. There are countless areas of human interest, and every one of them contains enthusiasts who have expert-level mastery of the subject matter.

Is it not reasonable for someone who was promised to be loved, supported, and honored all the days of their life to be invested in with the same energy that their spouse invests in other life activities?

I'm not here to tell you how to think. But I'm confident that you will find little marital satisfaction with someone who perceives you to invest more in playing poker and fantasy football than you invest in them. Because they will feel profoundly abandoned and neglected by you when you do. Ask me how I know.

○

If eliminating habitual invalidating response patterns in our relationships is the highest priority for reversing a trust-erosion trend so that we can learn how to have "successful" conversations with our partners (where both people feel better afterward—not worse), then the next habit I encourage people to work on lives under the umbrella term: consideration.

Another way to think about knowing our spouse or romantic partner relates to our ability to anticipate their needs as life is happening in real time. To not be frequently surprised by our partners expressing sadness or anger on account of something we never saw coming or failed to identify as a threat.

If my wife has a high-pressure business presentation coming up next Friday, is fighting a cold, and is grieving the loss of her grandmother with whom she had a really close relationship, then maybe the most effective way to communicate my love and support for my spouse is to make sure the kids, family pets, and—ESPECIALLY—me are not taxing her mental and emotional energy beyond their limits.

Perhaps I can be responsible for nighttime routines with the kids and running them to their extracurriculars and keeping the laundry moving so that my wife has time to prepare her presentation. Maybe communicating love and support can involve managing dinner and kitchen cleanup and any number of things to reduce the mental and emotional load on her.

I can talk with her. I can let her know that I see how much she's carrying—that I'm tuned in, connected, aware—and that I have her back. I can communicate that I'm paying attention to her calendar, and I can be mindful of the ways I might be able to adjust my own schedule to ease the burdens she's carrying, especially in life's most difficult and stressful times.

And this mindfulness can become a new mental habit. A new default setting that serves, rather than damages, our relationships.

In my real life, I would have just kept going about my business, waiting for my mentally and emotionally exhausted wife to continue to manage all of our lives as she usually did. Dinner plans. Laundry. Waiting for her to ask me to go to the grocery store or to think of something for dinner. Waiting for her to ask me to participate in house cleaning.

This is what it looks like to leave your partner alone in a marriage. This is what it looks like to be blind to invisible work that others do and to the invisible loads that others carry that allow us to live more comfortably at their expense.

## RELATIONSHIP SKILL #3: DIFFERENTIATING BETWEEN CHARACTER FLAWS AND HABITS

The great miscalculation in dysfunctional relationships is that pain is occurring because of someone doing hurtful things and that this person doesn't care about the harm they are causing nor about the people suffering as a result.

The hurt party believes they are being mistreated and that a good person would never hurt them this much, so the offender must be "bad."

And the accused party believes they are a good person who is NOT doing anything harmful; therefore, the hurt party SHOULDN'T feel hurt.

This toxic conversation can last forever if two people let it.

First, as we have covered, a good person can behave innocently and STILL cause harm. Accepting responsibility for doing or saying something that caused someone else pain is not the same thing as admitting guilt or agreeing with the implication that we did something "wrong" or "bad." It's simply acknowledging the very real truth that someone can feel pain as a result of something we do or say and that they don't need us to agree with them in order to feel that pain. Can we be the kind of people who choose to think, speak, and act in a way that indicates concern for the pain and damage that resulted from something we did or said?

I believe that we must.

Second, we can feel hurt by something that our partner said or did, and that action can have nothing to do with their character and everything to do with their habits and blind spots.

Attacking a well-intentioned person's character—or NOT taking care to word things in ways that communicate to someone else that we don't believe them to be bad people hurting us on purpose—is a sure-fire way to generate a defensive response.

And defensive responses invalidate. And invalidation always erodes trust. And trust erosion always leads to shitty relationships. And shitty relationships beget divorce and sad kids and future shitty relationships.

It's a vicious cycle that is in no way awesome.

It is useful for someone to recognize that they might be habitually, and accidentally, harming a person they love and care about without realizing it. It is useful for someone to recognize just how critical the conversations we have about this harm are to the success of the relation-ship. We don't have to drown in shame because we're not good enough. We don't have to wonder *What the hell is wrong with me?* We don't have to worry about being a hopeless asshole incapable of ever having healthy, loving, pleasant, connected relationships.

We must simply recognize that we have habits that inadvertently harm others, and then practice new habits until they take hold, replac-ing the accidentally harmful ones. It's a choice we make because the people we love deserve that from us.

And on the flip side, it's useful to look at our partners and think of them not as assholes doing asshole things but as people with different beliefs and different emotional experiences. It's useful to interpret the pain we feel not as the intentional behavior of selfish, narcissistic socio-paths (though I understand that a small percentage of the time that's what people are dealing with, and that it's not okay) but as the uninten-tionally habitual behavior of someone who hasn't yet learned a skill.

Helping our partners understand that things they can neither see nor feel are hurting us is useful. Using words and tones that might com-municate what worthless pieces of shit we think they are, is not.

We should not be married to people with poor character. And at the same time, we should be hypervigilant about making sure that our loved ones are not hurt because of things we're not paying attention to.

It always comes back to our mental and physical habits. This book can't help you become a better human being. And I would never sug-gest that you're not already a good one. But I do hope this book can help you think about the millions of little things you rarely pay attention to and consider whether paying attention to some of them might elimi-nate very real pain that your relationship partner—and you—endure as a result.

# RELATIONSHIP SKILL #4:
# ARGUING OR CRITICIZING EFFECTIVELY

We're human. So, avoiding conflict always and forever is an impractical idea. Even with the most considerate and lovable spouse imaginable, we are likely to find ourselves on opposite ends of an issue or to discover that we're disappointed with something they have said or done.

It's going to happen. The difference between an effective "argument" and an ineffective one, in my estimation, is whether we can maintain or even increase trust and communicate mutual respect despite our disagreement.

How might we do that? Fortunately, someone infinitely smarter than me already worked that out.

"*In disputes upon moral or scientific points,*" Arthur Martine counseled in his 1866 guide to the art of conversation, "*let your aim be to come at truth, not to conquer your opponent. So you never shall be at a loss in losing the argument, and gaining a new discovery.*"

**In other words, if you want to argue or criticize effectively, your goal can't be to win. The goal must be to arrive at truth.**

The goal, when offering criticism to someone else, should aim not to be right at all costs but to understand and advance the collective understanding, Martine said.

I think of it like this: Somewhere out there is the perfect combination of words and ideas that, if delivered at the optimum time and in the optimum way, will transfer information effectively from me to another person. Much of my writing and coaching work has more or less been me telling the exact same story in dozens of different ways, hoping one of them lands for someone. Sometimes they do.

Our partners will achieve clarity—full realization and

understanding—about the things we think and feel if we can find this magical combo of words and actions. Just as it's important for people to choose empathy and seek to better know and understand our romantic partners, we must also accept responsibility for tailoring our communication to its intended audience. How we address a classroom full of children is different than how we might address a group of incarcerated felons. Can we optimize our message for the person to whom we are trying to reach?

Here's a pearl of wisdom from philosopher and social psychologist Daniel Dennett's *Intuition Pumps and Other Tools for Thinking*, courtesy of Maria Popova's *Brain Pickings*:

### How to Compose a Successful Critical Commentary

1. You should attempt to re-express your target's position so clearly, vividly, and fairly that your target says, "Thanks, I wish I'd thought of putting it that way."

2. You should list any points of agreement (especially if they are not matters of general or widespread agreement).

3. You should mention anything you have learned from your target.

4. Only then are you permitted to say so much as a word of rebuttal or criticism.

A countless number of people—wives, usually—have reached out to me over the years with the question "What's your advice for how to get my husband to listen to me when I'm sharing my feelings or asking for help?"

Dennett's strategy for successful critical commentary is it.

## RELATIONSHIP SKILL #5:
## CONNECTION RITUALS

It's hard to be angry when you're laughing. It's hard to feel disconnected when your partner signals—verbally or otherwise—some inside joke that belongs to the two of you and no one else.

I believe a relationship skill worth developing and thinking about is the idea of having connection rituals. Very intentional actions or plans designed for nothing other than increasing the emotional connection and level of intimacy between two people.

One of my favorite connection rituals can't really be planned. It's a spontaneous occurrence initiated by one person in a relationship when they feel compelled to do so, and I have my stepsister to thank for teaching me it.

I call it The Peace Treaty.

One of the tools she or my brother-in-law use when they feel their temperatures rising during an argument is to leverage their mutual love of music and endearing immaturity to signal a peace treaty to the other in the middle of the conversation.

If they start to feel themselves getting angry and heading toward a blowup, it's not uncommon for one of them to say something like "Stop! Collaborate and listen," and if The Peace Treaty is working as intended, the other will respond, "Ice is back with a brand-new edition," singing the lyrics to Vanilla Ice's cheesy 1990 hit "Ice Ice Baby."

I like to imagine that some dancing is involved.

And for this longtime married couple, this type of exchange more often than not will lead to both of them laughing and making the very conscious decision to choose their marriage and one another over trying to score cheap debate or argument points in this particular conversation that is unlikely to matter even a tiny bit a day or week later.

This is a connection ritual. A powerful one. A private inside joke or code word or signal specific to two romantic partners that one can share with the other to say, *"Hey. What are we doing? I don't want to fight with you because I love you and I love us more than anything else. Whatever this is, we'll figure it out. But let's do it together. I'm on your side. I choose us."*

O

Yale Law graduate and former US Supreme Court clerk Gretchen Rubin (author of *The Happiness Project*) decided that feeling good mattered enough to research what helps people actually achieve it.

Some people quibble with the word "happy." I get it. It's a little bourgeois. We can use a more mature word like "content," if you prefer.

Regardless, the merits of pursuing feel-good things—be they substantial on some grand, selfless, serve-something-greater than ourselves mission; or perhaps something a little more indulgent like craving an orgasm, a fine whiskey, or a Snickers ice cream bar—will continue to propel human behavior, independent of how many of us might approve of any particular desire.

People don't like to feel bad. When things hurt, we will try to flee to safety. When things feel good, we'll bathe in it for as long as we possibly can until it's Monday-morning-esque end inevitably arrives.

In the simplest scientific terms, chemicals produced by our brains are what make us feel good. The three chemicals specifically linked to feelings of happiness are: oxytocin, serotonin, and dopamine. There are many ways to naturally (and artificially) get our brain to release these "happy chemicals."

One of the easiest ways is to simply prolong your hugs for a few seconds. Hugging for six seconds (not four, not five—SIX!) releases these chemicals in your body, and that of the person you're hugging.

Make that person your spouse. Your children. Other super-neat people that you love very much. Six-second hugs. Every day if you can. As often as possible if you cannot.

Six-second hugs. They're a thing. And another connection ritual we can implement if we choose to.

○

I was reminded of how egregiously I failed my marriage when I was introduced to the relationship habits of Jon and Missy Butcher.

Here's a couple that has been married more than twenty-five years, and instead of them complaining about one another to anyone who will listen like many of the twenty-five-year couples I've encountered, these two take a walk together every single day, as a daily check-in.

While most of us are busy holding in our frustrations so we can angrily spew them out in an undisciplined way at an inopportune time, the Butchers plan a time each day to meet, take a walk, and unload all of that crap to one another. They keep a daily appointment with one another to listen to the things the other had experienced earlier in the day, both good and bad.

This is what it looks like to intentionally move toward one another— to Move the Dots Closer, a key relationship skill and thought exercise we'll get to next.

Several couples I know have another powerful connection ritual— the once-per-week date night. Maybe at home. Maybe somewhere else. But every week, usually Friday or Saturday night, no matter where they are, belongs to them, and arrangements are made for everything else in their lives (children, pets, work) to be cared for.

This is their connection ritual. This is what it means to water your own lawn so that your own grass ALWAYS looks greener and better than whatever is on the other side of the fence.

Having a good marriage or a quality, connected romantic relationship of any kind is a lot like getting in good physical shape. A select few don't have to work very hard to look and feel great. But most of us do. And despite the efforts of many magic diet and supplement salespeople, there are no shortcuts to being our best selves physically.

We just have to do the work. And it's really hard at the beginning. Inertia is always the greatest obstacle. Something new is always more difficult to accomplish than something routine. Our first week of work is always more challenging and intimidating than our eighteenth month on the job.

We move every day. We are mindful about what we consume. The more we make healthy choices, the more our health and wellness benefit from those choices.

And so it is in our relationships. They are what the participants mindfully choose for them to be. When two people wake up every day making the choice to choose one another, and prioritizing one another over everything else, our connections grow. Our love flourishes. Our relationships thrive.

## RELATIONSHIP SKILL #6: MOVE THE DOTS CLOSER

Galileo Galilei and Isaac Newton's first law of motion—also called the "law of inertia"—states that a body or object at rest remains at rest and that a body or object in motion continues to move at a constant velocity unless acted upon by an external force.

Or, in regular-speak: If shit doesn't happen, nothing changes. At least that's how I always thought about it. If I set a lamp on a bedroom nightstand and never touch it, the expectation is that the lamp will sit still—right there—forever.

Applying that to my marriage, I believed stillness—inactivity or un-eventfulness such as going several days or weeks without an argument or negative incident—while not necessarily a positive, was at worst a nonevent. Harmless. Benign. Safe.

If my wife were watching something on HGTV in the living room, and I were watching basketball in the basement rec room, nothing was happening. Thus, in my brain, nothing bad happened.

I used to believe that Galileo and Newton's laws of motion didn't apply to movement within our human relationships but then realized I was the one getting it wrong. *Shock.*

The laws of motion absolutely apply to our relationships. My mistake was thinking of people in relationships as being inert, or still. If we were still, then nothing happening would be harmless. But we are not still. In our relationships, we are not at rest. We are CONSTANTLY adrift and, in my estimation, slowly drifting away from one another when we don't have a strong tether. It took me far too long to realize just how apt the metaphor "tying the knot" is.

And since a body in motion continues to move at a constant velocity unless acted upon by an external force, two people doing nothing AREN'T sitting still. They're drifting apart at a constant velocity until someone does something about it.

We are always either moving toward each other or away from each other.

Another way I think and talk about that is to Move the Dots

Closer. Imagine a horizontal line graph with two data points. One dot is you and the second dot is your significant other. Every day—every interaction—is an opportunity for those two dots to move toward one another or further apart.

While we're busy at work, distracted by our personal stresses, tasks, hopes, and dreams. While we're busy simply trying to stay alive, raise healthy children, keep our bills paid, etc., we are drifting away from our romantic partner.

A visual aid:

o————————o

Connected.

*A month later.*

o——————————o

Drifted apart a little.

*Three months later, after a great vacation, a nice anniversary dinner and gift exchange, mind-bending orgasms, and a job promotion for one of them, which alleviated financial stress.*

o———o

Boom.

*Four years later, after a new baby, a blown anniversary by the husband because ANOTHER promotion kept him super-busy and away from home a lot, five consecutive months without sex, and quiet avoidance of one another at home.*

o————————————————————————————————————o

On the brink.

If they continue to avoid the growing distance between them, they will continue to drift away from one another. The further they distance themselves, the weaker their connection—their bond—becomes, which then makes it vulnerable to outside forces (traumatic illness, a death in the family, sexual affairs, etc.).

O

**Every day—every conversation, every moment—is an opportunity to move closer to one another or further apart. You get to choose.**

Doing nothing is a death sentence. Because when we do nothing, we are NOT sitting still, biding our time waiting for something to happen. While we wait, we move apart. And I think couples—often men—are unaware of this constant, dangerous drift.

This is why focused, connected, mindful, present dinner conversations are so important. This is why six-second hugs are significant. This is why planning activities to do together—often and intentionally—is fundamental to the health of our relationships.

We are always moving away from each other. Always. So, we need to row our little boats against the current back toward each other often enough so that we're never too far apart. Tie knots. Tether ourselves to one another. Anchor ourselves to one another.

The goal of an emotional conversation with our partner can be to try to win debate points with them, while essentially shoving them further away. That's a choice we can make. Or maybe the goal of an emotional conversation with our partner can simply be to decrease the distance between the both of us. Maybe the merits of right versus wrong—the value of being "correct"—is a big, fat zero when it comes to our most important relationships.

Maybe the thing we should be measuring is the gap between us, constantly fighting to move toward each other.

O

We can wake up in the morning and make a conscious choice to connect. A kind word. A thoughtful action. While we are sitting at the office, hiking in the park, waiting in the lobby at a doctor's appointment, or standing in line at the grocery store, we can metaphorically move toward someone else.

*Maybe I can text her right now to let her know how important and beautiful she is. Maybe I can remind her today and every other day, how grateful I am for her to choose me and sacrifice for me. Maybe I can just check in and see how her day is going and if there's anything I can do to make it better.*

When we're tired after a long day at work or irritated by our unsympathetic children or in the middle of some home project we're doing—maybe we can strengthen our capacity for awareness, for patience, for mental discipline.

Maybe we can NOTICE the things in our lives that are All The Time. The "invisible" stuff we often look past and forget to feel grateful for. We forget to hug. We forget to nurture. We forget to love—not the feeling. We think and feel love but forget that other people don't always know what we are thinking and feeling. We forget to love—the action. People rarely misunderstand love the action.

The inevitability of doing nothing—of inertia—is a broken relationship. The inevitability is broken people.

When we're not moving toward one another, we're moving away.

Love is a choice.

Evaluating whether a conversation brought two people closer together or further apart is a skill that lives in the "rapport dimension" of communication, says sociolinguist Deborah Tannen, a Georgetown University professor and author of several bestselling books, including *You Just Don't Understand: Women and Men in Conversation.*

Tannen says that women, by and large, emphasize the rapport dimension in their conversations. They use conversation as a means of connecting with others—to build rapport with them.

Men, on the other hand, can often be observed as emphasizing the "status dimension" of communication. Tannen observed that men are often seen trying to score conversation points. To "win" the conversation by making a great point or by saying things designed to increase their own status in the eyes of others.

This is a profoundly important relationship skill. I don't pretend to know whether these tendencies are sociological or biological, nor do I particularly care. I do pretend to know that trying to win conversations almost always results in poor listening habits, mental and emotional invalidation of others, and, therefore, frequent trust erosion anytime words and ideas are exchanged.

It can't be said enough times: Erode too much trust, and your relationship is over. I don't believe we spend enough time each day aware of just how much our default thought and conversation patterns accidentally hurt people we care about.

## WHO SHOULD RANK #1 IN OUR RELATIONSHIPS?

Where should your spouse or romantic partner rank in your life? Take all the time you need to think before answering. Just please don't be a lying doucheface when you make your list as I would have been when I was married.

Ever have your wife ask you to fold a basket of laundry or clean up after dinner, and you said you would but then ended up playing video games all night instead? Unless situations like that are few and far between, please don't rank your spouse ahead of video games on your list.

Ever have your husband ask you to not complain about him to your mother or to please avoid discussing intimate details of your private sex life with your friends? Unless you did so as part of consulting those you trust for marital wisdom in the spirit of strengthening your marriage, please don't rank your spouse ahead of gossiping with your friends, mom, or whoever.

I think many—perhaps most—people have other things and people ranked ahead of their spouses. They won't say it. But they don't have to. We can see what people do. We can see what we do.

Ranking anything ahead of your spouse is the most surefire way I know to create mistrust and instability in a marriage that often leads to divorce and almost always unhappiness for everyone involved.

Here's how I think many married guys would publicly rank their Life Things (I'm intentionally leaving religious faith out of the conversation as it often proves to be an unproductive and distracting argument starter—though I think it's fair to note that I've never heard of a divorce resulting directly from two people putting their shared faith first and foremost in their marriage):

1. Marital Family
2. Family of Origin
3. Job
4. Friends
5. Favorite Hobby or Lifestyle Activity

But here's how I think many married guys actually prioritize their Life Things, according to their actions:

1.  Favorite Hobby or Lifestyle Activity
2.  Job
3.  Friends
4.  Family of Origin
5.  Marital Family

I worked hard to stop blaming my ex-wife for our divorce after she made the decision to leave. I used to get blog comments and private messages encouraging me to start shifting some of the blame to her. Something along the lines of *"OMG! Anyone freaking out over something as petty as a dish by the sink seriously needs to get her priorities in order!"*

The people who write and say things like that are missing the forest for the trees.

I don't like the word "blame." I don't believe relationship conflict is the result of people doing bad things. I believe relationship conflict is the result of people failing to understand and accurately calculate for how their partner will experience something they say or do (or fail to say or do).

Each message encouraging me to blame-shift toward my ex-wife appeared to me as someone who didn't understand what it means to accept personal responsibility, which is likely to result in them feeling like a victim every time something bad happens for their rest of their lives. Life is hard when painful things happen and we're helpless to combat them. It's only in accepting responsibility for our choices that we protect ourselves from perpetual victimhood.

If you insist that I share some honest criticism of my young wife back then, I would say that it sometimes felt as if my wife prioritized her family of origin over our marriage. I chose my wife over my parents if I had to rank them from a prioritization standpoint. And it never felt as if she did the same for me, though it's fair to point out that my behavior from the start may have never allowed her to feel safe enough to jump fully into a new nest that she wasn't 100 percent confident would still be there a few years later.

Later, it seemed as if she had doubled down by giving 95 percent of herself to our son once it became just the three of us. I thought I was being noble and unselfish by not calling it out, though in hindsight I'd already screwed up so badly at being a husband by that point that there's no intellectually honest or fair way to predict how she might have been after childbirth had I been effective at anticipating and fulfilling her needs.

*"But Matt! What about the kids?! Shouldn't they always come first?!"*

Nope. They shouldn't. And, as a father who loves his son more than anything else on this planet, I struggle writing those words. It twists my insides a little. **That's usually how I know something is true—when it feels uncomfortable and inconvenient.**

Prioritizing anyone or anything over your wife or husband is the most surefire way I know to destroy your family. In marriage, either our spouse is No. 1 or we are doing it wrong.

I say that without judgment. I'm divorced largely because I prioritized all kinds of bullshit ahead of my wife and our relationship. I offer it only as a thought exercise because I think most married people put at least something ahead of their marriage. And yes, that includes our parents and families of origin. And yes, that includes our children. And yes, that idea makes me uncomfortable.

But, it's still true.

"WAIT. Matt. Are you seriously saying we should choose our husbands and wives over our children? I can ALMOST understand the parents thing. But the kids? My kids come first no matter what!"

Do they really?

When we teach our children that they are the most important things in life and that if they want our attention they will always get it and that if they want or need something we always drop everything we're doing so that it is magically done for them and that the marriage between Mom and Dad isn't the top priority, what happens?

Bad news: You end up getting someone like me. (Sorry, Mom.)

You raise kids who grow up believing they're uniquely special even though they're not. You raise kids who lack self-sufficiency as well as self-awareness and who grow up expecting their partners to do things for them that their parents used to, but then also get mad at their partners anytime they feel as if they are being treated like a kid.

When we don't prioritize the relationship between Mom and Dad, we inadvertently raise kids who have no idea what a loving, high-functioning, healthy, mutually respectful marriage looks like. A marriage between two people who truly cherish one another and maintain their romantic and sexual spark through mindful intention and channeling energy into the human being they promised to love, honor, and serve for the rest of their lives.

The Adam and Eve Bible story famously depicts the first married couple. In the story, you'll find the word "cleave," which describes what we're supposed to do to our spouse.

The word "cleave" means "to adhere to, stick to, or join with." I think it's reasonable to assume the spiritual text is talking about a metaphorical bond of unity between them beyond promoting the literal act of inserting a penis into a vagina, but surely we can celebrate both the figurative and literal in this instance.

I don't get to tell people what to do. I don't think I have all of the answers and that you need my help. I'm not trying to communicate that I think I'm right about everything. You'll recall that my personal marriage data sample is both small and unremarkable and that my success rate amounts to abysmal failure.

But I still would like to encourage you to put your spouse first in your marriage and to encourage people to not marry one another until they're committed to the idea of truly putting one another first.

You'll be doing your girlfriend or boyfriend, their family and friends, and any children or pets you may one day share a huge favor.

Please remember: You don't have to get married, and maybe you shouldn't.

If your parents or siblings mean more to you than your partner, and you feel inside as if you'd choose them over someone you're considering marrying, then DO NOT get married. If your job or your friends or the fun things you like to do mean more to you than your partner, DO NOT get married. And [*big swallow*], if your children mean more to you than your partner, and you believe catering to their needs at the expense of your partner's is the right thing to do, then I think your marriage is a ticking time bomb. (**Note:** I'm writing specifically about married moms and dads who made babies together. I think it's both fair and proper for divorced or otherwise single parents to prioritize their children over people they're dating when there's still uncertainty about whether marriage is in the future.)

I caution people not to confuse LOVE with PRIORITIZING.

I can never love something or someone more than my son. That's unimaginable. But I can (hypothetically, in my sweet flux-capacitor-powered DeLorean) prioritize his mother.

As parents, we don't discipline our children because we somehow delight in upsetting them or taking away things that bring them joy. We discipline our kids to teach them lessons and to help them grow into better people with good values.

As a married or committed partner, we don't prioritize our spouses over children because we prefer to neglect the kids or show favoritism. We prioritize our spouses because it is what will help our children grow into better people with good values and provide a healthy model for how to succeed in their future relationships. Because if our kids are unable to navigate those, they're going to have challenges ahead that we as parents are ill-equipped to help with.

Physician Danielle Teller in "How American Parenting Is Killing the American Marriage," wrote, *"Children who are raised to believe that they are the center of the universe have a tough time when their special status erodes as they approach adulthood. Most troubling of all, couples who live entirely child-centric lives can lose touch with one another to the point where they have nothing left to say to one another when the kids leave home . . . Is it surprising that divorce rates are rising fastest for new empty nesters?"*

○

You're born to your parents. They and any siblings you might have are all you know and love.

Family by birth. Love tends to be a built-in feature.

When you're older, and your offspring are born, you are all they know and love. You're their everything. And the intense love we feel for our children is something beyond description.

But still—it's family by birth. Often, that love feels easy. We tend to not need any reminders to feel love for our kids.

But our spouse is something different. It's a particularly unique and special relationship. That's not inherited by birth or blood. Love is not some prepackaged thing that comes along with dating or marriage like it does with being born into a family or having kids of our own.

Our spouse is someone we CHOOSE. Out of every human being— billions of them—we choose that person. It is a love as rich and powerful as we have for our parents and children, but it's one that is grown. It's a garden we plant and tend. It's something entirely voluntary.

In marriage and relationships like it, love is a choice we must make every day.

More and more, people are coming to understand this but often not until their marriage is in shambles and they're trying to figure out why. Sometimes, like me, they don't come to terms with this until they're experiencing the aftermath of a painful divorce.

I didn't know what marriage REALLY was when I asked my wife to marry me or when I said "I do." The proof was in the pudding for the following nine years.

If more people entered marriage committed to this idea of putting their spouse first, and understanding why it's such an important mind-set, many more marriages would go the distance because they'd never deteriorate to begin with.

**You honor your parents when you put your spouse first.** You comfort them because they know you're safe and secure, and that their grandchildren are well cared for.

**You honor your children when you put your spouse first.** You teach them that they are, in fact, NOT the center of the universe and that the best way to live is to be aware of other people's needs. You teach them what marriage is supposed to look like. You provide a safe and unbreakable home. You provide a lifelong foundation for them on which they can anchor and build their futures.

**You honor yourself when you put your spouse first.** Because you are living for something greater than yourself and are less likely to die alone, sad, angry, and with herpes on your mouth.

Your parents will pass one day. It will be hard. You'll carry on because your spouse is always first and he or she will be by your side through the grief and transition. You will provide the same support for her or him.

Similarly, your children will move out one day. It will be hard. You'll carry on because your spouse is always first and he or she will help carry you through the loss and major life adjustment. You will provide the same support for her or him in return.

And there we will be. In an uncertain but tangible future if we're brave enough to choose it. Waking up every day seeking life-giving purpose and adventure. When we have wisely, courageously, spent the years leading up to this future putting our partners first, we won't have to look very hard to find either.

*The potency of this male-identity thing is the primary reason wives can't get their husbands to read relationship books, visit a therapist, or attend marriage retreats.*

# 7

# MARRIAGE AND THE MAN CARD

I MADE FUN OF MY GAY FRIEND IN HIGH SCHOOL FOR THE SAME reason I was afraid to tell my father and stepfather that I spent a bunch of time writing about relationships like some wannabe therapist following my divorce.

It's also the same reason I was a shitty husband and the same reason millions of men—even ones who are pretty good guys—are shitty husbands. Somewhere down deep, in places we don't like to talk about, most men are afraid of losing their identity as men. They're afraid of being rejected by their male peers. They're afraid of not being respected or sexually desired by women. They're afraid of disappointing their fathers, their coaches, their male mentors.

Men are so afraid of these things that we don't seek help when we need it in matters big and small, for fear of projecting a lack of "manliness." We sometimes won't even admit there's a problem.

*I can handle it! I'm a man!*

Men won't admit that they are bad husbands and fathers, even with all of the evidence in the world staring them in the face. Sad, angry, emotionally bent and broken wives. Jacked-up kids with daddy issues. Feelings of shame, dealt with in silence and pretend stoicism. We grow our shame piles but hide them behind masks. Behind alcohol and behind sex and behind work and behind escapist video games and behind a whole bunch of pretending to be happy while feeling something else.

Our pretend tough-guy behavior drives our wives and girlfriends away. The people we secretly hope will rescue us. We act like all we want our partners to do is placate our egos and sexuality. But this is just what we think we want. We are afraid of being honest about our emotions, about feeling uncertain or scared. We continue to run away from these fears and cover them up in wanting to be right, liked, and attractive—in the process often behaving in ways our partners experience as unlikable and unattractive. They are unable to constantly feed us what we want, and the relationship becomes a one-way street, a dead end. Our partners for the most part feel just as messy and needy as we do but they are honest about it. They are desperate to connect and not just go along for the ride.

So, we feel even more shame. *You did this to me*, thinks the broken, damaged man who feels like he gave up his old life for her.

*I was happy. I felt good. People liked me. I had friends. My life was amazing. And I gave up virtually all of it and promised you forever, and all you do is treat me like a failure every day. As if I'm a constant disappointment to you. As if you're so perfect and amazing, and I'm some loser piece of shit. And now you want to pin our shitty marriage on ME?! Go to hell.*

But he knows she's a little bit right. The proof is in the shame we feel. There's no shame when we have given all that we could.

The shame is the proof that we're guilty.

○

I attended a small high school in a small Ohio town in the mid-1990s. We played football and called things "gay" when we meant "stupid" and called each other "fags" as a slang bro-out locker-room put-down.

So, when one of the kids in our class exhibited voice inflections and hand movements we associated with being less than manly, some of us guys made fun of him behind his back. Because he was obviously gay, which was obviously the worst-possible thing to be because it meant you weren't a REAL man like us.

By the time senior year rolled around, he had suffered silently and mostly alone for the lack of acceptance he felt from many of us. He was a student leader on a retreat that many of my classmates attended that year and admitted during a speech in front of everyone that he had considered killing himself several times.

This guy who had NEVER—near as I could tell—mistreated me or anyone else was so uncomfortable at school that he thought being dead might be better than being around for what many say are the best years of our lives.

You might say I contributed to almost killing a kid in my class. An awesome and kind kid.

And it wasn't because I disliked him. I was never mean to him in any obvious or direct way. It was because I wanted to be acknowledged by my friends as a "man" while we cracked private jokes about him—signaling to one another that we were all on the same manly team.

That was more important to me than treating a good person with respect and dignity.

But, hey. At least I had my Man Card.

○

The potency of this male-identity thing is the primary reason wives can't get their husbands to read relationship books, visit a therapist, or attend marriage retreats. This male-identity thing from which I also suffer. Even today, if I'm not paying enough attention and operating on my default setting, I can be part of the problem.

## MEN WON'T SEEK HELP TO AVOID THE APPEARANCE OF WEAKNESS

I feel as if many Americans suffer from something I'll call *America Is #1, You Foreign Losers!!!* Syndrome.

You can't look around with intellectual honesty and say that all things American are somehow demonstrably better than things we observe in other countries and cultures.

In fact, it's nonsense. We have data available to anyone with internet access that proves that other countries are better at [insert public policy of choice here]. Some places have more successful schools. More effective transportation. More thriving economies. And, it pains me to say, but maybe even people who, as a whole, are infinitely more pleasant to be around than, as a whole, a random same-sized sampling of people in the United States.

My favorite example of *America Is #1, You Foreign Losers!!!* Syndrome is learning that US students are pretty middle-of-the-road at math performance but lead the world in being confident regarding their math skills. .

The Brown Center Report on American Education, which sets out to gauge how well American students are learning in school, discovered, for example, that the least-confident eighth-grade math student in Singapore still outperforms the most-confident American eighth-grade math student.

In other words, American students think they're awesome at math, but they're actually a little bit shitty.

Sound familiar? I don't blame these students for their potentially misplaced confidence. Confidence is mostly a good thing. When your default setting, however, is certainty in your own goodness or correctness or smartness or capability, the reality is that you're fallible in all of those areas. And then the likelihood of fuckery is especially high.

If I'm a good person AND I'm smart AND I'm nice AND I'm married? I'm a good husband, I concluded.

Men are confident in their abilities as husbands and fathers or, at the very least, demonstrate confidence by actually getting married and actually fathering children. And it's because they're a lot like American math students. They're not actually good, but they think they are, or at least are damn sure going to tell you they are. Like a man.

It starts to get ugly when wives who want emotional honesty from their spouses have experienced the inevitable danger of trust erosion. They then try to get their husbands to give more to them and their marriage or family. You can see where this is going.

*Oh, so I'm suddenly no longer good enough for you? I gave up my fun, single life for this? To be constantly reminded of my shortcomings and have you point out all of the ways I disappoint you? This is so unfair and is not what I signed up for.*

O

The world fails men. Specifically, boys.

We fail everyone, but we fail men in a way that correlates closely with miserable adult relationships and identity crises.

Perhaps documented most effectively in filmmaker Jennifer Siebel Newsom's *The Mask You Live In*, we have created "a culture that doesn't give young boys a way to feel secure in their masculinity, so we make them go prove it all the time," said sociologist Michael Kimmel.

This failure leads to a countless number of men—some incredibly smart, talented, strong, brave, and decent men—achieving positions of influence where they inevitably perpetuate the cycle of collectively failing men, and by proxy, the women and children in their sphere of influence.

Husbands. Fathers. Big brothers. Best friends. Business leaders. Celebrity influencers. Politicians. Coaches. Educators. Commanding officers. Group leaders. Classmates. Teammates and tribesmen.

What men in these positions think, believe, do, feel, and say affects countless people—the ripple effects of which can last for centuries. Many of these guys are amazingly virtuous. Many are trying their best every day to live according to the values instilled in them. They're simply following the examples of their male role models from their youth.

These aren't evil men muahahaha-ing and fist-bumping a bunch of other sadistic D-holes in the secret back room of their private male-only clubs. I mean, some are, but those dipshits aren't hard to spot, nor are their crimes dangerously undetectable.

What is so dangerous about the world failing men is that we've created billions of very decent human beings who unknowingly walk around every day trying their God's-honest best but are accidentally napalming their homes and closest relationships.

## LIFE WILL BE MEASURED BY OUR FAMILY AND FRIENDS—NOT ALL THAT OTHER STUFF

Life is essentially a contest to see who can have the most people say truthful, authentically nice things about us at our funerals.

Men are taught that status is everything. It's reinforced by women because women are often attracted to high-status men. It's reinforced by children because children's lives can often benefit in observable ways (financially and socially) from high-status fathers.

Men pursue wealth. Men pursue fame. Men pursue physical attractiveness. Men pursue business ventures, athletic competitions, and hobbies where they succeed. Men pursue sexual conquests. Men pursue the accumulation of material possessions. Men pursue all of this shit that doesn't mean a damn thing to ANYONE the second the doctor tells them they have terminal cancer or they discover their wife having an affair or try to digest their child's suicide note.

What people really want is to have PURPOSE.

And all of those aforementioned "successes" have a legitimate purpose in our personal lives. I'm not trying to trivialize success in personal ventures. It matters to all of us.

I'm saying that many of us coast through much of life unaware of this truth:

**The biggest influence on how good our lives are is the quality of our human relationships.**

No amount of money, possessions, career success, trophies on the shelf, notches on the bedpost, nor fame can provide the peace and contentment we all crave down deep inside.

Fear. Sadness. Pain. Anxiety. Anger. Stress. Grief. Shame. These are the mortal enemies of all of us, but surely of men. When we put those we care about, live near, and work with first—selfless love, humble leadership, principle above profit—the only life currency that actually matters starts to accumulate.

And then when we do that enough, more people will cry and share funny stories at our funerals instead of not giving a crap that we croaked because they kind of thought we were assholes anyway.

Much of what we believe about marriage and relationships as we enter them is wrong. It's not our fault. It's our responsibility, of course. But not our fault. All we have to go on is our parents, who either divorced or fumbled through marriage hiding most of the hard stuff from us because they weren't taught any of this either.

Our marriages or long-term relationships (or lack thereof) ultimately prove to be the biggest influencers on our day-to-day lives. **If our relationships are shitty, our lives are shitty.**

○

I spent the years following my divorce dissecting my failed relationship from every angle I could, asking *What could I have done differently that would have led to a happier result for my wife, son, friends, and extended family?*

If my divorce were someone else's fault, then that means it's a lottery. Dumb luck. It means I am a helpless victim to the passing whims and fancies of whomever I date or marry and have absolutely no control over what happens to me or my son.

But if I'm responsible for my personal life turning out as it has— *and I am responsible*—then there's hope. I don't have to be afraid of it happening again.

My marriage ending was the worst thing that ever happened to me. There is no close second-place thing.

One morning when I was dropping off my then third-grader at school, he told me that he doesn't like Mondays because no matter which of his parents he just spent a fun weekend with, he knows he's not likely to see them again until Wednesday evening and that it makes him feel sad.

As a child of divorce myself, I think a lot about what that boy has had to carry because of me.

Someday, maybe even while reading this sentence, he'll realize that his father failed his mother and, by proxy, him. He'll realize that choices I made resulted in his life feeling shittier and more difficult than necessary. Because of all of the times I chose myself over his mother.

Living this way can ruin us. Poison us. Break us.

Broken people raising broken children. Broken fathers raising broken sons. Broken men raising broken boys and girls who don't always learn how to be whole again. Girls who may never learn what it's supposed to look and feel like when a husband loves a wife. Boys who may never learn what it looks like to love and serve our families, to lead humbly, and how the rewards of unbreakable marriage and family are much greater than the short-term highs of their individual pursuits.

Boys and girls become the new men and women. And then they don't teach their sons the things they needed to know. So, the boys grow up repeating the sins of their fathers.

Not because they're bad. Just because they didn't know better. Because their parents didn't know. And their grandparents didn't know. And neither did anyone else.

Marriage is difficult, and everyone "knows" it just like we know that fire can burn us.

And yet, we often end up learning the hard way as our relationships crumble around us just like we can only feel the intense pain of severe burning in the middle of the fire.

And too often, for a long time afterward.

# MEN ARE 300 PERCENT MORE LIKELY THAN WOMEN TO KILL THEMSELVES

I kept my writing a secret from my parents and most people I know until media coverage forced me to disclose it.

I kept it a secret from people like my mom and grandma because I was afraid of them reading my locker-room profanity or my hinting at immoral sexual fantasies when I was newly divorced and on a celibacy streak only clergymen and famous virgin celebrities can appreciate.

I kept it a secret from people like my dad and stepdad because I didn't want them reading that I used to cry a lot after my divorce or that I had begun to question so much about the male behavior that had been modeled for me growing up or to discover the fact that I was now someone who spent much of his time thinking about, talking about, and writing about relationships. You know—"girl stuff." You know—so they didn't think their son was some candy-ass wimp.

○

The fear is real. And it's the same fear many men you know hide behind their veils of stoic machismo. Even though women are more likely than men to report suicidal thoughts and tendencies, men are statistically three times more likely to kill themselves.

This phenomenon, this gender paradox with suicide, is observed in every race, culture, religious affiliation, and country in the world.

*Why?* Because men don't want to lose their Man Card. It's something we joke about with friends, but when we feel as if we actually lost it because our wife left us or because we're losing our hair or because of erectile dysfunction, a job loss, or difficulty keeping our bodies looking the way we want them to as we age?

We're afraid to seek help. Because that's tantamount to admitting weakness or that we're not man enough. The only people who can understand are OTHER men equally disinterested in advertising to their male peers just how dark and lonely it sometimes feels inside our own heads.

So, most of us don't say anything.

And then when shit really hits the fan? With major financial problems or health issues or the loss of our marriage and family? That noose or gun trigger after a bender starts looking like a viable escape plan for broken men.

In Will Storr's "Why Men Kill Themselves in Such High Numbers," which ran in *Pacific Standard*, Storr highlights how certain societal and cultural norms drive men to vigilantly fight for this often-elusive sense of manhood:

"Even in the developed world, where gender equality is not as bad as in developing countries, most men still see themselves as being responsible for providing and protecting their family. Of course, some women are social perfectionists too. But men's social perfectionism is much more harmful.

"'A man who can't provide for the family is somehow not a man anymore,' said Roy Baumeister, a psychology professor at Florida State University. 'A woman is a woman no matter what, but manhood can be lost.'"

O

Men could use help in the mental and emotional health space as much as anyone can use help with anything. But we refuse it because we don't want to believe that we need it or are terrified of what it says about us that we DO need it.

We'd rather appear strong, even if it's a facade.

So, we accidentally destroy our marriages. And we accidentally ruin relationships with friends and family.

If it makes us feel shame, or feels like something in which we can't succeed, we turn around and walk the other way, but we make sure it looks like something manlier than fear.

We never just say, *"For the same reason I don't know how to design rocket engines and navigation computers for space shuttles, I also don't know all there is to know about how to feel great about my life and have successful relationships with my wife and kids and friends and self."*

But I wish it felt safe to. Or better yet, even when we're afraid, I hope we'll have the courage to.

## THE TAXONOMY OF MARRIED MEN

**TAX·ON·O·MY**–noun–\tak'sänəmē\—the classification of something

O

Here's the breakdown:

1. **Husbands.** All husbands fall into one of two camps, which for the purpose of this exercise, require defining.

**GOOD MEN.** A good man is the kind of person you'd let spend the night in your house without hesitation. A good man can be trusted to care for your children and pets. A good man is generally kind, honest, reliable, respectful, polite, and loving and demonstrates loyalty and commitment to his family, friends, co-workers, teammates, etc. A good man is not perfect. But his Pros in the character department far outweigh his Cons.

**BAD MEN.** A bad man does not care how his actions affect others. He hurts people physically and emotionally without remorse. He cons people to take advantage of them. He lies. Cheats. Steals. Rapes. Murders. Abuses. He is toxic to himself and everyone around him, and his toxic behavior is intentional. His behavior can legitimately be described as evil. He revels in chaos, drama, and dysfunction. He takes pleasure in others' pain. A bad man is a constant danger to himself and anyone near him. His Cons far outweigh his Pros.

Let's not waste much thought on bad men. I lack the maturity and patience to explain to a stranger who is unlikely to be reading this or to ever care what I say why knowingly marrying, or intentionally remaining committed to, a BAD man is a shitty life decision.

2. **Husbands Who Are Good Men.** All good men who are married fall into one of two camps.

**GOOD HUSBANDS.** A good husband performs the duties of marriage with skill and competence. His success is usually most apparent to his wife, who feels loved and secure most days of her life and who loves and respects him in ways she's only ever felt for her children and her very closest family members. He is often appreciated by his in-laws, admired by his friends and neighbors, secretly or not-so-secretly wanted by women who covet the things he provides his wife and family in their own lives, and has very little conflict-related drama or life stresses at home with his wife and family.

**BAD HUSBANDS.** A bad husband is shitty at marriage. No matter how GOOD of a human being he is, he sucks at the complexities of human relationships. (**Note:** This puts him in the 95 percent of everyone who at times struggles with the complexities of human relationships. This does not make him stupid or incompetent or unfit necessarily for anything good men are suited for. It just makes him bad at marriage. Throughout human history, good men have been bad at many things, like singing and dancing or constructing high-rise buildings or playing the piano or carving ice sculptures or solving advanced mathematics.)

I am not going to waste thought and space here on men who are good husbands. They're awesome. I appreciate them. I hope you do too. Let's talk about bad husbands.

3. **Good Men Who Are Shitty Husbands.** All good men who are bad husbands fall into one of two camps.

**MEN WHO DON'T KNOW THEY ARE BAD HUSBANDS.** Either these men don't know they're bad husbands because they don't know what shitty husband-ing is and/or no one has ever taught him that he's one OR anytime someone (usually his wife) says that he is, he doesn't actually believe it. (**Note:** I believe, of all married men in existence, the VAST majority—I'm talking 85-ish percent—fall into this category.)

**MEN WHO KNOW THEY ARE BAD HUSBANDS BUT WANT TO BE GOOD.** This is a very bad spot to be in because, to arrive here, one usually has to have a miserable, failing marriage wreaking so much emotional havoc, stress, and anxiety in our home lives that we FINALLY decide to ask ourselves the right question: *What can I do to help fix this?*

Now that we have a common understanding of the classifications, let's dig deeper.

○

One night at dinner, my wife said, *"I don't know if I love you or want to be married to you anymore."*

I reacted poorly and made it entirely about me. I pouted and started sleeping in the guest room, from which point every day got a little harder and more difficult over eighteen months before she chose to move out and end our relationship. But months before she left for good, something in me snapped. I wanted to—*needed to*—understand why this was happening.

I knew that I loved my wife. I knew that I wanted to stay married. And I thought that, because I was a good man, and because we shared a son, our entire adulthoods, a home, and many friends, we should be able to pull through.

*All you need is love! Right? RIGHT?!?!* Wrong.

Just like being a good man and being a good husband can be mutually exclusive things, so too can love exist in the shittiest and most painful marriages.

○

One night, I found myself reading the book *How to Improve Your Marriage Without Talking About It* by Patricia Love and Steven Stosny, two longtime marriage counselors who used their experiences with clients and years of note-taking to explain common marriage problems and how husbands and wives often experience them.

The experience of reading about random married couples who were having identical conflicts and conversations as we were had a profound effect on me and set the stage for the fundamental shift from who I was to who I am.

Here's what my brain did afterward:

### REALIZATION #1

*Wow. Our problems are so common that generic, made-up stories in a self-help book totally NAIL my marriage. These exact same marriage problems are affecting almost everybody.*

### REALIZATION #2

*If these relationship problems are this common, that means my wife and I aren't somehow fatally flawed. We're not NOT soul mates or freaks unfit for marriage. These problems are practically universal and we don't have to feel ashamed for having them.*

### REALIZATION #3

*If nearly all marriages suffer these common problems, then that means it's foolish to get divorced with the intention of replacing your spouse with someone else. Because these same problems will ALSO exist with that other person. If my wife and I love each other, our son, and both generally prefer marriage to being single, the most logical course is to work hard on this marriage rather than trying to start new relationships as middle-aged, divorced, single parents only to inevitably have to work hard on THAT relationship, but with the added suck of all the family and friends breakage and losing so much time with our children.*

○

I was too little, too late. It was painful to realize that what was done could not be undone.

You don't want to be the guy trying to save his family while his spouse has checked out of the marriage because she's been beaten down emotionally so much through the years while he—a genuinely good dude who simply sucked at marriage—didn't realize it.

And now he KNOWS. Now, he *gets it*. But his partner is done.

Few relationships come back from the dead. It's a difficult pill to swallow.

Yet the value of understanding where we went wrong, how to avoid being shitty husbands in the future, and how to teach our children to have healthy and functional human relationships can't be overstated.

First, we took Husbands, and split them into two groups—Good Men and Bad Men.

And this isn't about "nice guys" versus "bad boys." Nonconformist "bad boys" engaging in mischief with sometimes aggressive, daring, and tough exteriors can still be very good men. We're talking about character. Not personality type.

Women are often attracted to men who do bad things. But good, healthy people are not attracted to BAD people. I'm comfortable saying that people should NOT marry, remain married to, or have children with fundamentally bad people.

So now we have Husbands Who Are Good Men, and we're splitting them into two groups—Good Husbands and Bad Husbands.

Lots of good men are lousy husbands. Being a husband is a skill. Just like playing instruments, flying helicopters, and performing heart surgery. A very good person can be bad at marriage. It's an important distinction. Good husbands can't benefit from anything I ever think or write, so we're homing in on Good Men Who Are Bad Husbands.

○

We split them into two groups as well: The ones who don't know they're bad husbands (which I guesstimate to be about 85 percent of all married men) and the ones who DO know and are trying to be better (which mostly include men on the brink of losing their family, and in their desperate search for answers, realize as I did that they'd been accidentally messing up for many years).

I'm operating under the assumption that no GOOD man could KNOW he's a bad husband and intentionally refuse to alter his behaviors. Because that would make him a bad man.

Conclusion: Troubled marriages worth saving only involve good men.

I'm probably biased. I—perhaps delusionally—think of myself as a "good" man. I'm not always nice. I don't always do the right thing. I certainly upset people now and then. But I know who I try to be and I'll share a humanity foxhole with anyone else trying to be this way too.

I'll go to bat for these husbands and fathers over and over and over again if they demonstrate the humility and effort required to evolve on behalf of their wives and children. And many men will.

The powerful influence of simple awareness in our lives can't be overstated. People are willing to change when they understand why change is needed.

Most men who repeatedly hurt their spouses simply don't know why the behavior changes are needed. A good man armed with correct information changes the entire world for his marriage and family. Beautiful things. Hero shit. And we should all be doing more of that.

# ACCIDENTAL SEXISM RUINED MY MARRIAGE (AND MIGHT BE RUINING YOURS)

Here are the top two definitions for the word "sexism." One of them applies to me and one does not:

1. prejudice or discrimination based on sex; especially discrimination against women

2. behavior, conditions, or attitudes that foster stereotypes of social roles based on sex

I did, said, and believed things throughout my youth and marriage that were totally sexist—even though I didn't view them as sexist at the time—and those things more or less turned my wife against me and ultimately cost me my marriage and family.

If you'd have told me I was a sexist, I'd have undoubtedly responded with defensive outrage and mansplained how you were wrong, all the while believing everything I was saying and feeling.

That's the real danger. THAT is what causes all of these relationships to slowly turn ugly and then end miserably—that we 100 percent believe all of the bullshit we peddle. We're telling the truth. We act like we're right and as if we know everything because we all actually believe it at the time.

Life's worst things happen while we feel certain about things that aren't true.

○

It doesn't matter that I didn't believe I was sexist. What matters is that I was a sexist.

My mom more or less ran the household growing up with her and my stepdad and was the alpha regarding parenting decisions about what I was allowed or not allowed to do, or to determine punishments when I was maybe not being awesome.

Most of my teachers were female.

The two very best students—the most intelligent and top-performing kids in my class—were female. I think both are doctors now.

I had close-knit friendships with a few of the girls in my class that at the time rivaled my close friendships with guy friends.

All of this to say that I never believed that men were fundamentally better than women.

## FEAR PERPETUATED MY SEXISM— IS IT THE SAME FOR YOU?

I never disliked someone because they were from Iran or Saudi Arabia or Pakistan. I've always liked pretty much everyone, which is very ENFP of me. (My Myers-Briggs personality type.)

But in the aftermath of September 11, 2001, I was afraid— irrationally—that someone from a particular ethnicity was somehow more likely to harm me than someone who looked like Timothy McVeigh (who in 1995 blew up the federal building in Oklahoma City, killing 168 people) or Mark Barton (who in 1999 shot twenty-five people, killing twelve, after having murdered his wife and children two days earlier).

I think we can agree, in hindsight, that my fear of being harmed by someone on account of their skin pigment was a pretty stupid thing to believe.

O

Where I came from, it was BAD to be a guy who did anything like a girl.

As recently as my twenties, I was giving major judgy side-eye looks to buddies who listened to Taylor Swift ("girl music") or who liked watching romantic comedies ("chick flicks").

It wasn't bad to be a girl. It wasn't bad to be a woman.

It was simply bad to do things "like a girl" if you weren't one. We were all little homophobic assholes. We spent so much time calling each other "gay fags" as a way to rip on one another that we were clueless of the impact it was having to those around us. There's no chance that any of the kids questioning their gender identity or sexuality or who actually were gay could have ever felt respected, accepted, or comfortable around us. We didn't think we were bullies. But we were bullies, and I regret those actions and the impact they must have had on the people around me.

The societal norm where I grew up was clear: If you're a man who does "girl things," you're less of a man. Which is bad.

It seemed a given that women do the majority of housework, the majority of child care, the majority of social calendar management, etc. There was no right versus wrong judgment about any of it. It was just The Way. It felt normal.

And we, as human beings, tend to treat things outside of OUR idea of normal as being "wrong."

## IT WAS MY WIFE'S RESPONSIBILITY TO FIX HER DUMB EMOTIONS, I THOUGHT

*If my wife were responding incorrectly to things because she had weak girl emotions, how was that MY fault?*, I thought, conflating my wife's individual thoughts and feelings with my own brand of sexism.

*Is it really fair to ask me to adjust everything I do, think, feel, and say simply because it hurts my wife's incorrect feelings when all she has to do is realize her mistake and simply STOP feeling bad about silly things?*

After writing about marriage and divorce for several years, I've come to believe that the above sentiment is among the top marriage killers in the world. It's an invisible, quiet belief that triggers the Invalidation Triple Threat response pattern, regardless of gender.

I ALREADY did more around the house than every male role model I'd ever had.

I was ALREADY compromising my Man of the House role and was hell-bent on retaining my Man Card.

I was working and making the most money. I was doing more housework ("women's work," you might have heard it called) than any of the adult men I grew up around. I didn't do drugs or drink excessively. I didn't gamble away our savings. I wasn't physically or verbally abusive. I was a reliable caretaker for our son.

So, whenever it seemed as if she were telling me what an insensitive and shitty husband I was being, my reaction was always one of defensiveness and high-and-mighty moral outrage.

*How DARE you tell me I'm not a good husband!*

O

"Matt, would you please stop throwing your jeans on this nightstand? I try hard to keep the bedroom looking nice. Can you please just put them in the closet out of sight?"

*How DARE she make a big deal out of something stupid like throwing my jeans on the nightstand that literally no other human being besides us will ever see! Why make a marriage fight out of this small thing?!*

○

*"Matt, would you please stop leaving that dirty glass by the sink? I try hard to keep the kitchen looking nice. Can you please just put it in the dishwasher?"*

*How DARE she make a big deal out of something stupid like setting that water glass by the sink that isn't even dirty! I'm just trying to recycle the glass because it's easier than washing extra dishes every time. Why make a marriage fight out of this silly thing?!*

○

*"Matt, would you please not make fun of me in front of our friends? It hurts my feelings. You're literally nicer to total strangers than you are to me."*

*Oh my God. How DARE she make a big deal out of something stupid like some playful mocking that everyone knows is a joke! I married this woman and chose her out of EVERYONE IN THE WORLD to love and commit to and have children with! Why make a marriage fight over this totally illogical thing?!*

○

I loved my wife. But I didn't RESPECT her individual experiences as being equally valid to mine.

Things that were real and true—and often painful—for her didn't affect me. Not outside of her complaining to me about it. My wife spent many years trying to recruit me to understand what was happening in her heart and mind so that I would work cooperatively with her to eliminate negativity in the marriage.

She tried every way she knew how to communicate to me that these issues she was bringing to my attention were important. Each and every time she tried, I made it clear to her how much I disagreed and how certain I was that I was correct (by virtue of my wise man brain).

This idea can't be shared enough times:

My wife HURT—down deep where the medicine can't fix it—because of things I said and did. And for more than a decade, when she came to me for help to make the hurt stop, I communicated to her that I thought she was mistaken—even wrong—to feel hurt.

I believed her failure to take responsibility for her emotions was the primary problem in our marriage. I seriously said that to her.

Every chance I had to respect my wife and live up to the vows I'd made on our wedding day, I instead communicated to her: *No. Your feelings are dumb. It's not MY job to stop doing these things that don't even matter. It's YOUR job to stop caring about them so that you won't feel hurt anymore.*

This is why my wife could no longer trust me or feel safe with me. When you don't behave in a manner that results in your partner feeling safe, you eventually lose their trust, and then it's all over.

○

Men lie constantly. I think maybe everyone does.

Sometimes, they are classic bald-faced lies: *"I didn't do it!"* Even though we all know he did. Sometimes, they are exaggerated lies, like when basketball and football players' heights and weights are inflated slightly.

And sometimes, the lies are so subtle and nuanced that most of us don't even think of them as lies. There is no malice in the deceit. The deception is not to harm others and, in fact, may be to preserve another's feelings: *"No. Seriously. I think you look beautiful with your super-short haircut!"* Even though he thinks it's boyish and unattractive.

There are also many other deceitful moments that might seem harmless as they're happening, and as isolated incidents, probably are. But they're not isolated. They're constant. Not "constant" in a hyperbolic way. "Constant" in a That Guy Is Wearing a Mask and Hiding Fundamentally True Parts of Himself from Everyone way.

*Why?*

He wants his Man Card. Even if it kills him. He wants it to be good enough for his father. He wants it so he can feel accepted by members of his various tribes—friends, sports teams, fellow soldiers, professional networks, fraternities, hobby groups, social clubs, etc. He wants it because he believes it will make him attractive to women.

There's The Man Way® to do things. And all things must be done that way *because I'm a man, not some wussy little girl! I'm doing it The Man Way!*

And it's a little bit funny because there's no universally established Way Men Do Things.

Everything depends on culture, environment, and behavior models. It's not uncommon to see two heterosexual male friends holding hands in public throughout the Middle East or South America—a sign of respect in those places that many of us throughout the rest of the world might not consider at first glance to be "manly" behavior. Where I'm from, you'd almost never see guys wearing pink, and rarely purple, when we were growing up. Those were "girl" colors. But now, it's not only common, but fashionable, to wear pink or purple shirts and neckties.

In other words, The Man Way is a constantly moving target and purely dependent on where a guy lives or the specific culture of a group to which he craves admission or acceptance.

Take beer drinking, for example. Some guys are strictly Budweiser guys. Hell, maybe they even want it canned. And they're going to drink ten to twelve Budweisers because *Real Men drink a lot of beer!* And don't you dare try to give him some fancy-boy craft beer like he's some uppity hipster or metrosexual.

But then other guys are strictly craft beer guys. And maybe they only want draft beer in a pint glass. And they're going to drink like a refined connoisseur, and if you want an education on beer styles or brewing techniques, this Renaissance Man will tell you all about them. Don't you dare try to give him some cheap-ass swill like Budweiser. *Only cretins drink piss like that.*

But maybe the Bud guys will play along and drink stouts and IPAs in a crowd of craft beer drinkers, and maybe Craft Beer Guy will pound Budweisers out on the boat or golf course with his friends on a hot, sunny day.

And maybe they'll be just a tiny bit dishonest about their real feelings in an effort to fit in.

It happens all the time. Probably with everyone, every day.

But when it happens with men because of the Man Card thing, our relationships suffer.

When our relationships suffer, the rest of our lives suffer. We take more damage that we brought on ourselves. And then the even-more-damaged versions of us repeat the cycle, but it only gets worse.

We wonder why. Because *we're MEN. Strong. Logical. Correct.*

*We're not little emo girls who sit down to pee, hit from the red tees, drive wimpy cars, play with smaller basketballs, go to the restroom in groups, or do girly things like cry and talk about our feelings.*

Men get indignant. *No one tried to feminize our fathers and grandfathers! They fought wars and built things with their hands!*

O

Our identity has so many stakeholders, we believe.

Our parents and extended families. Our friends. Our romantic partners. Our kids. And everyone we interact with. And sometimes we're not who we really are. We're who we think we're supposed to be for everyone else.

I think this is a root cause of many divorces.

The social skills "acceptable" for women to showcase are the life skills required to avoid shitty relationships, full of fighting, dysfunction, infidelity, sexlessness, or every other horrible thing couples suffer from before their eventual divorce.

Divorce damages men HARD. Harder than women, all the experts say, and there are a million reasons why, but the main one is this: As a general rule, wives do way more for marriages and families than men do, so when a marriage ends, it's harder for a man to maintain his way of life because he can't replicate nearly as many marriage tasks she performed as she can of his. And that's just the logistical side.

Within ourselves, another war is raging. The idea of who we think we are versus the reality of our failure as a husband and/or father. We are not honest with ourselves from the beginning. We suppress rather than vulnerably share and understand our emotions. Then the finality and clarity of this lost identity leaves men with nothing to hold on to.

We're left with a terrifying question that only our choices moving forward can answer: *Who am I, really?*

In my estimation, women are demonstrably BETTER—more skilled, more knowledgeable, more capable—at relationship skills than men (due to culture and socialization norms, not biology).

And since I can't think of anything more influential or important to our daily existence than our relationships, the conclusion is simple:

Male behavior is mostly responsible for the divorce crisis; thus, men are the key to solving it.

## SOLVING IT WILL REQUIRE REDEFINING MANHOOD

Men get pissed at me all the time. They read one of my blog posts shared on Reddit, or linked in some online forum, and the message is always essentially the same.

*"I'm tired of everyone blaming guys for everything! Look at you turning your back on your gender and pandering to women! What a simp! Look at all these women showering praises on you, but I bet if you wrote about all of the things they do wrong, they'll tell you what a sexist pig you are! The writer of this blog needs to clean his vagina, because his ex-wife clearly took his balls with her when she left! Women are the real problem!"*

I pity them, along with their wives, girlfriends, and children. Because that guy has no chance. Not in his current form.

I mean, he might find a subservient wife to cater to his every whim and suffer in silence. He might find a trophy wife who appreciates his substantial wealth and enjoys those financial luxuries without him while he's away on business. He might find a physical or emotional punching bag to make him sandwiches and give him on-demand oral.

But I don't think that man can ever have what I perceive to be the foundational thing we need for a life of contentment—one where we enjoy being alive and don't feel miserable every waking second of every day: stable, healthy, loving, reliable, energy-giving relationships.

**And as long as men collectively believe that The Things You Must Do to Have Healthy Relationships are "girl things," then I think heterosexual marriage is doomed.**

If communicating effectively with our partners about the things we think and feel is a "girl thing," and, therefore, bad so we won't do it, then we have no chance. If sacrificial love and a willingness to compromise or be influenced by our partners' wishes is a "girl thing," and, therefore, bad so we won't do it, then we are screwed. If courageously taking off our masks that hide our real selves from everyone else and protect us from imagined rejection and judgment—if being truly vulnerable with our partners—is a "girl thing," and, therefore, bad so we won't do it, then maybe we deserve this fate.

Because the only way to kick ass in your relationships is, in many respects, to play "like a girl."

And if we're going to be too much of a wimpy bitch to accept that? Well, I guess we'll always have our armchair where we can rot slowly before dying alone, marinating in loneliness and anger while marveling at how young we looked in that faded Man Card photo.

*Never put your girlfriend or wife in the position of having to do things for you that your mother did for you when you were growing up at home.*

# 8

# SHE FEELS LIKE YOUR MOM AND DOESN'T WANT TO . . .

YOUR MOM PROBABLY DOESN'T WANT TO HAVE SEX WITH YOU.

I work hard at not judging because, glass houses and whatnot. But that's a good thing, right? Your mom not wanting to sleep with you? Because eww?

For this conversation, the genesis of the whole don't-bang-family policy is less important than simply understanding that it's a thing. Most people are not sexually attracted to their parents, siblings, children, etc. in the same way that they ARE sexually attracted to whomever they end up attracted to later in life.

Here's why this idea matters for your present-day sex life: If you are a man in a marriage or romantic relationship and your wife or girlfriend is performing functions for you that are identical or similar to things your mother did for you (or their mother did for them) in childhood, she will eventually start to feel like your mom and stop wanting to touch your penis.

Some of you might be thinking *But Matt! That's bullshit! I know women who love taking care of the men in their lives by ironing their shirts or serving them a cold drink after a long day at work! It's because they love and appreciate their husbands!*

Neat! I know people who prefer eating cold, rigid, unmelted cheese slices on their hamburgers, and I think they're savages. Different strokes and stuff.

Many of us know women (and men) who exhibit a servant's heart. They routinely demonstrate love through acts of service for others—one of Gary Chapman's famous Five Love Languages—and this can sometimes manifest as a wife or girlfriend who derives pleasure from serving others, including her partner. These voluntary acts may include cooking, cleaning, folding laundry, packing lunches, etc.

Just as there are people who prefer playing basketball to basket weaving or who spend their leisure time hunting and fishing instead of going to jazz clubs or crafting googly-eyed popsicle stick figures.

I prefer to avoid saying things I can't back up with data, but I'm comfortable predicting that the vast majority of women—just like men—feel that scrubbing toilets, folding and putting away laundry, and scheduling doctor's appointments for children are shitty jobs and they wish they had a magic fairy to do that work for them.

I'm being totally serious here—the best sex advice I could ever offer a young person entering a long-term romantic relationship is this: **Never put your girlfriend or wife in the position of having to do things for you that your mother did for you when you were growing up at home.** Turns out, this is in no way an aphrodisiac.

To be clear, it's cool if your wife or girlfriend does these things voluntarily or because after thoughtful conversation you both agreed to structure your relationship in such a way that she routinely performs these household responsibilities.

Problems arise when our behavior communicates to our partner that they MUST do this work because it's EXPECTED of them. People (usually wives and mothers) perform these thankless, joy-sucking tasks with no acknowledgment or gratitude for their sacrifice.

Domestic household work is often referred to as "invisible"—work that is being done, or must be done, with people like me paying too little attention to notice. Also, "invisible" because it's unpaid labor, which people value less than work that brings income into the household, even though domestic housework and child care are, in my experience, more difficult and frustrating than any of my professional jobs have ever been.

In marriage or a long-term relationship, things get messy when there is little to no effort on the part of one of the spouses or partners to recognize that these things are difficult and shitty.

In a male-female marriage where the guy is showing up as I did in mine, it appears as if he doesn't care to ease the burden for his partner by mindfully, proactively participating in the planning and execution of some of that work. If he did, he not only eases the burden of shared responsibilities but she feels seen and recognized for her contributions—contributions that allow us to live the less-burdensome lifestyle that we do.

It's about respect. Children tend not to respect or feel genuine gratitude for the many sacrifices their parents make in an effort to provide them food, clothing, shelter, educational and social opportunities, etc. Most of us forgive children for this oversight since we were all children once, and we acted the same way.

But when an adult partner behaves as children do? It tends to lessen (read: deaden) sexual desire in their partner as one might expect of a healthy adult's physiological response toward a child.

And since a healthy sexual relationship is a pillar on which lasting marriages are built, when one spouse starts responding physically to the other as they might in a parent-child relationship, things can go south rather quickly, and I mean that in a way that has nothing to do with oral.

I've heard a lot of frustrated guys vent to me about how little their wives want to have sex—as if she's weaponizing it or punishing them. These guys think they're the exact same guy she chose to marry, thereby blaming her for "changing."

"*She never wants to have sex!*" they say.

Not quite, my friend. She just doesn't want to have sex with YOU. It hurts because it's true.

If you're guessing that this condition is a common recipe for extra-marital affairs, you just won a delicious imaginary cookie. A common affair scenario stemming from the She Feels Like Your Mom situation looks like this:

A stressed-out, underappreciated, emotionally neglected wife and mother of two spends the majority of her life working forty-plus hours per week at a day job, only to come home and have to manage the lion's share of household tasks (the Mental Load) AND have to perform most of them, else they never get done. No one says thank you. The kids and her husband frequently undo whatever nice thing she just accomplished (cleaning floors, wiping pee dribble from toilet rims, rinsing toothpaste from bathroom sink basins).

Kids run off to play with their friends and participate in school extracurriculars. Husband runs off to hide in his man cave or tinker outside in the yard or garage or stays away from home altogether to play golf or have after-work drinks with his friends.

*"Why doesn't my husband want me or want to be around me?"* she wonders.

Maybe he comes home from the bar and grabs his wife's ass and tries to bang one out while he is buzzing from the alcohol and reacts angrily to his wife's cold disinterest or rejection. Or maybe it is less gross than that. Maybe, with total respect, he expresses interest minus the un-invited handsy stuff, and she declines in a polite way because she has had a difficult and exhausting day. And even though he politely responds that he understands, he feels a deep sting of rejection from a wife who seems to be growing increasingly more distant and disinterested in him.

Maybe at work, some handsome fella in corporate accounting is thrown onto a small project team with the wife, where they are tasked with solving a company problem together. Maybe after several work conversations and long hours together, the handsome fella says or does something to demonstrate how attractive he finds his female co-worker.

He listens respectfully to her input and ideas. He admires her intelligence and project management skills. And without being a creeper, he is smitten by her smile, the way her eyes sparkle when she laughs at his jokes, the way she rocks those business-casual office outfits.

When the man at home for whom she does everything and to whom she has pledged her entire life totally ignores her, never wants to spend time with her, never says thank you for folding his laundry or picking up after him, and never speaks or acts in ways that communicate how attractive or sexually desirable she is . . . well, that's what people in the bourbon industry might call the perfect mash bill recipe for making Your Wife Totally Wants to Orgasm Several Times with Her Handsome Co-Worker straight Kentucky bourbon.

I don't know what percentage of women in this situation would act on those desires and engage in an affair, but I'd like to submit the idea that it doesn't much matter.

Even if your wife or girlfriend never actually sleeps with this guy, she wants to. She WANTS to! Only fear of the consequences or a disciplined personal code of conduct is stopping her.

Serious question: Do either of those physical affair-stopping behaviors make you feel any better about her actually WANTING to? That she might close her eyes and think about him instead of you when you are in bed together or that she would rather touch herself in the bathtub thinking about him than be touched by you?

○

In my viral blog post "She Divorced Me Because I Left Dishes by the Sink," I wrote a paragraph that gave a bunch of male readers heartburn: "*But I remember my wife often saying how exhausting it was for her to have to tell me what to do all the time. It's why the sexiest thing a man can say to his partner is 'I got this,' and then take care of whatever needs taken care of.*

"*I always reasoned: 'If you just tell me what you want me to do, I'll gladly do it.'*

"*But she didn't want to be my mother. She wanted to be my partner, and she wanted me to apply all of my intelligence and learning capabilities to the logistics of managing our lives and household.*

"*She wanted me to figure out all of the things that need done and devise my own method of task management.*

"*I wish I could remember what seemed so unreasonable to me about that at the time.*"

This does NOT mean, every day of my life, that my wife bossed me around. It does not mean I awaited her daily instruction on how I could be her manservant, catering to her every whim, as a bunch of dudes imagine as some emasculating horror show they seem to think I'm advocating.

My wife was awesome about keeping our house clean and organized. She always performed 70-ish percent of every house chore (including back when we were dating). More importantly, she MANAGED tasks (took on the responsibility of thinking of what needed to be done and how it would be done) closer to 90 percent of the time.

Like many adults today, we both grew up watching our moms do most of the housework while our dads went off to work and mostly stuck to "man chores" like mowing grass, shoveling snow, sanding and staining decks, cleaning the gutters, taking out the trash, etc.

Because I wasn't as self-aware in my youth as I am now, I didn't identify the imbalanced workload that wives and mothers typically carried.

My wife, often on Saturday mornings, wanted to clean the house. I would have been happy to wait an extra week or two because I don't like cleaning in the same way you don't want to bang your parents. But I wasn't going to sit around watching SportsCenter while my wife scrubbed toilets, vacuumed floors, dusted furniture, and wiped down bathroom vanities. Not even I was that big of an asshole.

The house chores discrepancy became magnified when we brought our baby boy home from the hospital. If you're anything like me, those initial days and weeks were surreal, and every moment as a new, ill-prepared father was spent thinking, *What the hell do I do now?*

My wife wasn't like that at all. She wasn't like me. She had talked to other moms and prepared herself for some of the challenges of caring for newborns through reading books and online research. She wasn't any more ready to be a parent than I was, but instead of putting her head in the sand and hoping everything would magically work out, she took the initiative to make sure our home, and she as his mother, was as prepared as she could possibly be.

I wasn't asking my wife to boss me around.

But I was asking my wife to help me help her. Once again, I was asking my wife to not only do most of the work around the house, and with our newborn child, but I was also asking her to MANAGE all of those tasks. If she didn't remember to do something herself, or to ask me to do it for her, things didn't get done.

It was the most stressful time physically, psychologically, and emotionally my wife had ever been through. The health and well-being of her and our little son rested entirely on her being the best mother possible. And instead of putting in the work to support those efforts the best I could, I totally abandoned her to do all of the baby work alone while I sat around daydreaming of the future, when I would be throwing the football around with him in the backyard. We totally do that now too. My son and I, and it's great. But instead of mom watching from the deck with a drink and a smile, she has a new mailing address.

○

Many sons grow up hero-worshipping or at least modeling behavior after their fathers. Dad watches sports on TV and does "man chores" and maybe makes most of the money, if we're thinking of the old-fashioned models consistent with my 1980s childhood.

Mom cleans and folds their clothes, vacuums their bedroom, replenishes the refrigerator and pantry, cleans their pubic hairs from showers, washes dishes after dinner, and packs lunches.

But mom has an even-harder job.

Mom often manages the schedule for every member of her family. Not just for herself but for her children's school, medical, and extracurricular needs; her pets' veterinarian appointments; and then her husband's stuff too.

It's hard to be an adult sometimes. Even when you only have yourself to worry about. But it is especially difficult when you're managing logistics for sometimes uncooperative children as well.

If you want to toss a little piss mayonnaise on an already rancid shit sandwich, choose to be the kind of adult who focuses exclusively on your own needs and leave your adult partner to fend for themselves, your children, AND you. See how that works out for you.

Men (not all men—just too many) demonstrate great capacity for derpy-derping around waiting for their wives or girlfriends to provide some type of instruction. One of the greatest gifts you can give your romantic partner is to alleviate them of that burden—the burden of being IN CHARGE of shared household responsibilities, and perhaps sparing them any self-congratulatory behavior after picking up the kids from school or scheduling your own dentist's appointment.

Invest the time and mental energy necessary to understand what needs done, how it needs done, when it needs done, within your household, and take proper care of any children and pets you might have. Don't leave YOUR things for your spouse to take care of. It will accidentally happen sometimes, but when it does, SEE that it is happening, acknowledge it, and share your sincere appreciation for it.

If I had to distill the problems in failed relationships down to one idea, it would be our colossal failure to make the invisible visible, our failure to invest time and effort into developing awareness of what we otherwise might not notice in the busyness of daily life.

The alternative is to believe that shitty marriages and divorce are the results of intentionally relationship-damaging behaviors. Most people are not out there purposefully inflicting pain on their loved ones with the hopes that their relationships will soon end.

How is it possible that good people accidentally hurt each other this much?

Because it's invisible to them. Even when their partner tries desperately to communicate what they're feeling. The damage, and the events that caused it, remain largely invisible to one or both people.

So much of my work today is about helping others "see" what may be hiding in their blind spots and how to effectively navigate conversations during these potentially painful moments when conflict arises when we're not careful. That can look and feel like a subtle act of disrespect from a delayed response to a text message or an insensitive remark about a new haircut, or it can look and feel like wholesale rejection of who someone is.

*"How can he think I'm THIS stupid or THIS crazy or THIS weak or THIS unfair, and actually feel authentic feelings of love and respect for me? How is it possible for someone to genuinely love me but still hurt me more deeply and more often than I've ever been hurt before?"*

We routinely invalidate our partner's experiences when their thoughts and feelings don't align with ours. But the worst of us (and by "us," I mean this massive group of Good People Who Are Bad Spouses) twist the knife further by failing to actively participate in our relationships.

We don't invest time, effort, and energy into our relationships that would eliminate nagging concerns about how much our partners feel loved, supported, respected, desired, appreciated, etc. We don't invest time, effort, and energy that would result in our partners TRUSTING that we are a safe, healthy, reliable choice to spend the rest of their lives with.

We don't listen actively when they share concerns, fears, frustrations, hopes, and dreams. The thoughts and feelings that matter most to them often go in one ear and out the other, or we react to them in some thoughtless way that invalidates whatever we just heard.

And then there are our observable actions.

We are often—routinely—more polite to friends, co-workers, and even strangers than we are to our spouses. We often demonstrate great interest in things—work, sports, politics, fitness, video games, texting with friends, and countless hobbies. And because we demonstrate authentic interest and active participation in these things, it's quite obvious to our partners that we're NOT showing interest in them as people nor showing interest in shared activities—whether those be pleasurable activities or shared domestic responsibilities.

If you're anything like me back when I was younger and shittier at marriage, you may have never considered the idea of sexual attraction and desire being linked to life things like child care or pet care. You have maybe not considered that someone's feelings of being loved and desired—even in a sexual way—could be linked to noticing that a load of laundry needs folded or plans must be made for dinner or that there's a massive extracurricular family calendar for couples and their children, and being left to manage that calendar alone can consume and exhaust people.

This conversation extends far beyond sexual appetites and attraction. Shared household responsibilities (child care, dinner, housecleaning, bill paying, pet care, lawn maintenance, social calendar and extracurriculars, etc.) may very well be the greatest cause of relationship conversations that turn into fights. Shared household responsibilities surely generate Invalidation Triple Threat conversations as much or more than any other subject.

Eve Rodsky's excellent book *Fair Play* explains these relationship dynamics in a way that really landed with me. In *Fair Play*, Rodsky gives a shout-out to sociologists Arlene Kaplan Daniels and Arlie Hochschild, who in the 1980s coined terms for these "invisible" conditions that routinely tear relationships apart from the inside out.

"No doubt you too have read articles describing this 'mental load,' 'second shift,' and the 'emotional labor' that falls disproportionately on women, along with the toll this domestic work takes on our lives more broadly," Rodsky writes. "But what are we really talking about here?"

We'll break it down this way:

## THE MENTAL LOAD

The Mental Load refers to the invisible but massive and constantly fluctuating to-do lists we all have in our heads. Managing this mental to-do list is one of my greatest personal weaknesses, even when I'm only worrying about me and my schedule.

In marriage and long-term romantic relationships, there are other people's to-do lists (partners and children) to worry about as well. I really sucked at that part.

Stress, anxiety, and fatigue are pretty much a foregone conclusion. Rodsky mentions forgetfulness as well. Forgetfulness is often the reason people's feelings are hurt by well-intentioned partners, friends, and family members. Forgetting a birthday or an anniversary can be the most innocent act of one's life, but the other person can still feel profoundly hurt due to their apparent invisibility and evidence that we prioritized a bunch of other things over them.

## THE SECOND SHIFT

It's common for an adult (commonly women in male-female relationships) to perform a number of unpaid tasks in the mornings before heading to their job and then again when they get home from their day at work. Dinner. Dishes. Bathing children. Packing school lunches. Scheduling doctor appointments. Laundry. Walking the dog. Cleaning bathrooms. Vacuuming floors. Dusting surfaces. Grocery shopping. And so much more.

This is the recipe for producing exhausted adults who have little time for, and little interest in, sex—especially if it has to be with a partner who seems to forget they exist and who routinely abandons them to do thankless Second Shift work alone while they run off to work out, play video games, or watch television. And then remembers his partner exists only when he wants to touch her in bed. At this point, sex with this person feels like another joyless, thankless task on the Second Shift to-do list.

## EMOTIONAL LABOR

Coined by Hochschild in her 1983 book *The Managed Heart*, the term "emotional labor" has evolved over the past four decades to include "maintaining relationships" and "managing emotions," notes Rodsky, ". . . work like calling your in-laws, sending thank-you notes, buying teacher gifts, and soothing meltdowns [by children while shopping in stores]."

Emotional Labor can extend to the idea of a sad and angry wife remaining silent about what she's thinking and feeling for fear of upsetting her husband while he's trying to relax at home after work. It can extend to being responsible for a couple's entire social calendar—planning get-togethers with friends, parties, vacations, and holiday travel.

This work does not always fall exclusively to women in hetero couples (or just one partner in same-sex couples), but I think we can all be adults here and admit that—even two decades into the twenty-first century—that's exactly what happens most of the time.

## INVISIBLE WORK

Rodsky refers to "invisible work" as "the behind-the-scenes stuff that keeps a home and family running smoothly, although it's hardly noticed and is rarely valued."

Stocked food pantries. Folded clothes in dresser drawers. Clean bedroom sheets. Acquired school supplies. Veterinarian appointments for pets. Holiday and seasonal home decor. You get the idea.

Wives and mothers nod their heads, while dudes the world over say *What?! It's not like that stuff is hard, and I'm happy to help out whenever she asks me to as long as I'm not busy watching the ball game or playing first-person shooter video games!*

○

If you're interested in touching your naked partner more often than you do, there may be no quicker path than eliminating childlike irresponsibility and increasing your capacity to accomplish tasks to free up time and energy for your partner.

While we are on the subject, let's talk about the idea of "duty sex."

## DO SPOUSES OWE PARTNERS SEX?

Are married people obligated to have sex with their spouse?

Because the word "owe" isn't limited to legal, enforceable, or contractual obligations. It's also defined as "to be under a moral obligation to give someone something."

The most-fair question I can think to ask is this: In instances where two people marry in good faith, sincerely pledging sexual faithfulness to one another for life, could it be said that they have a moral obligation to fulfill one another's sexual desires?

The concept of "wifely duties" is typically rooted in traditional religious values about wives submitting to their husbands. There's a better-than-average chance you've attended a wedding or church service where you heard it mentioned. It gives every champion of human equality heartburn, and I imagine it's incredibly uncomfortable for women (and possibly some men) who've been abused in the past by a domineering tyrant. I grew up attending church on Sundays, have never been abused by a domineering tyrant, and it STILL makes me uncomfortable.

I'll let law experts weigh in on the legal definition of the word "owe." But how about in the general sense of the word? I suppose if someone's wife or husband promised it verbally or in writing (and ideally while *wanting to*, and not out of obligation), then maybe she or he would "owe" him or her the way I "owe" my mom a phone call when I don't call her often enough like a good son.

But the real heart of the matter is this: Do wives owe husbands duty sex by virtue of their marriage? Or vice versa?

Are wives or husbands "morally obligated" to sexually relieve or satisfy their husbands' or wives' urges?

The answer is no, regardless of the many reasons. What if she has the flu? What if his best friend died that day? What if the family pet needs taken to the emergency vet? What if she ran a marathon in the morning and says she's too tired? What if he didn't get much sleep because of a sick child? What if she or he had a rough day at work and simply isn't in the mood? Or, what if she just doesn't want to?

Remember the famous John F. Kennedy quote: "*Ask not what your country can do for you, but what you can do for your country*"?

Great quote. Applies to marriage. Marriage is NOT about what it can do for you or, more specifically, what your partner can do for you. Author and speaker Seth Adam Smith might have said it best in his viral blog article "Marriage Isn't For You."

Marriage is about what YOU can give to your marriage. It's about how YOU can make your spouse's life better. I feel comfortable saying that **unwanted sex NEVER makes someone's life better.**

How do we become more attractive and desirable to our partners so that they WANT to be intimate with us?

It's obvious to most of us that when two people who promised one another sexual exclusivity and faithfulness stop wanting to have sex with one another, a problem arises for either or both partners with a sex drive.

But most people don't truly understand WHY this happens. I think most people believe "*That's just the way it is! Everyone goes through this!*" or that it's the other person's fault (maybe!) or that the two of them simply "fell out of love."

It is less complicated than that but a hell of a lot more nuanced.

I believe most of us enter marriage totally unaware that what made us attractive or desirable to others as young, single people are not the same traits that our long-term relationship or marriage partners will find attractive later in life.

In other words: All of the shit you did that resulted in your partner wanting to go to bed with you back before you were married becomes mostly ineffective in long-term relationships.

What do I mean? Let's talk about it.

**Your physical appearance.** No matter how physically attractive you are, no amount of rugged good looks or a chiseled physique can overcome feelings of mistrust and danger a person might feel as a result of relationship insecurity. This goes back to Maslow's hierarchy of needs model. After air, food, and water, we require safety to live healthy lives. Single people we dated in our youth didn't feel unsafe or foster feelings of mistrust because they hadn't experienced emotionally painful or trust-betraying moments with us yet. Serial killer Ted Bundy was famously handsome. Actor Zac Efron (another dude people swoon over due to his looks) was tapped to portray Bundy in the 2019 Netflix film *Extremely Wicked, Shockingly Evil and Vile.* I'm confident that few, if any, would consider Bundy an ideal husband or father given his propensity for murder.

**Your bank account and status.** Money is attractive because it represents both safety and opportunity. Money provides long-term financial security that people crave as well as the resources to join the ranks of high society and engage in attractive lifestyle activities (travel, fine dining, exclusive social groups, etc.). But if our partner feels unsafe BECAUSE of our relationship, no amount of commas and zeros can offset the pain and fear of feeling trapped in an unhealthy relationship or living with the gnawing sense that the relationship and lifestyle are unsustainable.

**Your "game."** Confidence only works when it is authentic. Humor and intelligence only work when kindness and trust are present. And while mind games or deception might work for bar pickups and one-night

stands, dishonesty—or even just the lack of an authentic connection between two mutually trusting and vulnerable people—will eventually end
a marriage or long-term romantic relationship.

○

Sometimes I look at the search terms people type into search engines
to find my blog. On more than one occasion, I ran into the following:
*"magic potion to make a woman crave for sex."*

I laughed too.

But then I found myself thinking about it because it's a conversation
topic with merit.

If people assume (as I naively did for years) that their partners generally experience sexual thoughts and activities in the exact same ways
that they do, it's no wonder there is so much dysfunction, cheating, and
crappy relationships happening.

Put another way, your partner leaving you because of your inability
to understand how leaving dirty dishes by the sink can erode trust and
inflict emotional harm would be essentially the same thing as them
leaving you because of your inability to satisfy them in the bedroom.
(**Hint:** It would have almost nothing to do with your bedroom skills or
the quality of your performance.)

My anonymous friend stumbling on my blog during his digital quest
for magic sex potion is highly unlikely to ever read this. But maybe
someone else will.

## HOW TO BREW MAGIC SEX POTION

There's actually a way to elicit sexual desire from your partner without
magic, my funny Googling friend. And it's a pretty useful thing to know.

### Ingredient No. 1–Listen Actively and Understand the Ideas They're Sharing

When I unscientifically polled my Facebook audience regarding the biggest frustrations and pain points in their relationships, the top answer was "active listening." Many romantic partners (women, most commonly) report painful, dissatisfying one-way conversations with their significant other. Put plainly, MANY women in long-term relationships with men feel an absence of intimacy and emotional connection between them due to their partner's apparent disinterest in conversing with them. Don't read this as a "needy" wife not getting her way.

Active, engaged conversation is one of the most common ways humans connect and build trust with one another. Thus, a husband's or wife's reluctance to participate in meaningful conversation is often interpreted as disinterest and rejection.

*"He literally doesn't care about what happened to me today, or what I'm concerned about tomorrow. It appears as if he could spend every day of his life not knowing what I think about, what I do, what I feel, nor why. He simply doesn't care. That's how little I matter to him."*

Do your partner's stories bore you sometimes? LISTEN ANYWAY. This potent Magic Sex Potion ingredient is less about your organic interest in the conversation's subject matter and more about your mindful, intentional decision to participate in conversations covering ideas that matter to your partner. It's the ACT of sharing this time and exchanging ideas that grows intimacy between two people. You might move from boredom to very interested if you actually make the effort.

**STEP 1**–Be quiet and listen to your partner tell their story or verbalize a problem they might be having. Try hard to not interrupt unless it is to ask an engaging question that moves the story forward and demonstrates active listening and mental investment.

**STEP 2**–Don't sigh and act disinterested. Don't ask whether the story has a point. Don't behave as if everything they just said was dumb or otherwise not worth your time and attention. And for the love of God, if you're a guy dating or married to a woman who is sharing her frustrations about something personal she's dealing with, **DO NOT TRY TO SOLVE HER PROBLEM WITH YOUR MAN-SUGGESTIONS unless you are specifically asked for advice**. You're making a small-time investment like you do when you work out or like when you save money for retirement. You are investing in your partner's well-being and security. It might not make sense to you that something as seemingly meaningless and passive as just sitting there and listening can make your relationship profoundly strong. But it can, and will, if you just take a deep breath and, with love and respect, listen.

**STEP 3**–Enjoy how it feels when your partner respects and appreciates you and tells their friends and family how great you are. Enjoy how it feels when she wants you to ravish her instead of fantasizing about her project partner at work or the furnace repair guy.

## Ingredient No. 2–Be Vulnerable

Being vulnerable must not be confused with acting weak. This is not advocacy for weakness. Vulnerability is about being strong enough and courageous enough to share our truest selves with someone else even when we're afraid of rejection. There's nothing weak about it. It takes enormous strength and courage to share our deepest thoughts and feelings because it's the REAL US, instead of pretending as if we think and feel whatever we believe they want to hear.

Also, vulnerability is a form of honesty. And honesty fosters trust. A failure to be vulnerable is akin to hiding true things, which will always erode trust. We must preserve trust at virtually any cost if we want our relationships to remain healthy and strong.

### Ingredient No. 3–Be a Leader

This does not mean "dominate." This does not mean acting as if you are intellectually or emotionally superior or "in charge."

*"I'm the man of the house and you will respect me, damn it!"* I'd think not in a gross, sexist way, but certainly in an entitled way that might have seemed gross and sexist to anyone paying attention.

I couldn't even be trusted to adequately care for the house, the children, the pets, or even myself (per the norms of my marriage) for a long weekend if my wife were to leave town for a getaway with friends or her mom.

So, it's funny to me now how I thought I was so awesome and deserving of her unrequited respect and lusty desire.

Being a leader means:

- We accept responsibility for the quality of our marriage or long-term relationship.

- We accept responsibility for the behavior and "success" of our children.

- We accept responsibility for hurting our partner's feelings even when we don't understand how or why it happened.

- We accept the challenge of not repeating those behaviors.

- We do not passively ask our partner to manage the entire household's calendar and make every decision about food or weekend activities, only to complain when it does not align with our preferences.

- We accept responsibility for making our partner feel sexy and desired, planting the I-Want-To-Have-Sex-With-You seeds at unexpected times throughout the days and weeks. It's not their job to do us on demand. It's our job to be someone they want to do it with.

## Ingredient No. 4—Prioritize Your Partner and Never Stop Dating

If you are legitimately disinterested in the person you decided to commit the rest of your life to and share resources with, what in the hell are you doing? And why?

Date your partner. This isn't about feigning interest in them. It's about authentically demonstrating it.

Asking better questions always yields better answers. Ask questions. Ask why. Actively seek to better know and understand your partner. Their likes and dislikes. Their interests. Their fears. Their hopes and dreams. And listen to the answers.

When we have mastery of who our partner is and what they want, we can participate effectively in them pursuing their best life. When we don't know or don't care? We become an obstacle in their individual pursuits of happiness. If that happens, they will not only stop wanting to sleep with us but they will stop wanting to know us.

## Ingredient No. 5–Exercise

Exercise is sexy and attractive, but for reasons I'd argue are far more important than toned arms and a flat stomach. Those things are gravy.

Exercise demonstrates:

1. Self-respect.

2. Discipline and follow-through, which demonstrates consistency and trustworthiness. And lastly, actively demonstrating discipline and follow-through creates within you . . .

3. Confidence. And confidence—not the kind we fake, but the kind we organically exude because we authentically feel it—is sexy and attractive.

**Directions:** Combine all ingredients. Serve immediately, forever.

○

Regardless of your gender or preference, sex can be a powerful force for both good and bad in relationships, my potion-seeking friend. We've only scratched the surface.

*Many—maybe even most—relationships that deteriorate do so in part because we avoid discussing private, vulnerable thoughts and feelings for fear of judgment or rejection.*

# 9

# SEX, LIES, AND INTERNET PORN

**NOTE:** IF YOU GAVE BIRTH TO ME, ARE RELATED TO ME, REMEMBER me as a polite young man from church, attended school with me, worked with me professionally, dated me, or otherwise know me personally, you might want to skip this chapter.

○

Sooooo. I've totally masturbated before.

Maybe once. Or maybe 87 million times. Truthfully, I don't want to talk about it because it makes me really uncomfortable, and I can't stop thinking about my mom or grandma reading this and saying *"Heavens to Betsy! Did you know that Matt played Diddle-Me-Elmo?!"* nor can I stop imagining everyone I knew in high school sitting around going *"Ha! I knew it! I totally knew that guy wanked it!"* followed by them making plans to announce it at our next high school reunion.

It kind of makes me want to set myself on fire. But that feeling is why I'm talking about it, because we can't talk about relationships and marriage with intellectual honesty if we pretend that pornography and masturbation aren't actually things.

They are things.

Because pornography content companies tend to be privately held, it's difficult to get precise numbers for how much money the porn business generates.

An *NBC News* report in 2015 (the most recent data I could find) estimated the global porn industry to be worth $97 billion. That same report estimated that the United States alone accounted for $12 billion of that, which at the time, made porn more influential than Hollywood, Netflix (about $11 billion each), and pro basketball (the NBA earned about $7.5 billion).

The implications of that $12 billion US figure are extraordinary. What that means—the US porn industry being worth $12 billion—is that, statistically speaking, EVERY American, including newborn babies, nuns, and ninety-year-old grandparents, spends an average of $40 annually on pornography, even though there is basically limitless free porn on the internet.

Conclusion: You've totally wanked it, too, you little Pervy McPerversons! Don't worry. It'll be our little secret.

Many—maybe even most—relationships that deteriorate do so in part because we avoid discussing private, vulnerable thoughts and feelings for fear of judgment or rejection. This fearful reluctance to share ourselves honestly results in our partners believing things about us that aren't true.

It's difficult to have trust when one or both of us don't know the truth. And without trust, everything falls apart. Not sometimes. Always.

## SEX AND SECRECY

For the first decade of marriage, Miranda never really knew who her husband was, sexually, though she believed she did.

Peter was, by all appearances and reputation, of exceptional character. Tall. Handsome. Clean-cut. Kind. Shy. Reserved. Innocent. Sexually pure. A virgin until age twenty-nine.

He was running for public office when they met. Miranda, inspired by their shared political ideology, joined his campaign staff, and fell in love with him.

Peter was nothing like the other men she had known and dated. He seemed like a bona fide good guy, and after a few past run-ins with men who weren't especially good guys, she admired and fell in love with this disciplined man who chose principle over pleasure and wanted to help people more than he wanted power.

A gorgeous, red-haired, green-eyed bombshell not physically dissimilar from the animated Jessica Rabbit character from the 1988 film *Who Framed Roger Rabbit?*, Miranda turned heads in whatever room she walked into. But Peter's head seemed to always be focused on his mission. Like a boy scout, minus the badges and neckerchief.

*Peter is such a remarkably good guy,* she thought. *I'd love to spend the rest of my life with someone like him.*

While the campaign fell short of winning the election, it proved to be an incubator for Peter and Miranda's relationship. With the election behind them, they could date without any conflicts of interest, so when Miranda finally expressed her desire, the shy and reserved Peter said yes.

Their first kiss lasted more than an hour. A torrid, passionate romance began. The couple had an active, seemingly healthy sex life.

Peter had just one sexual encounter prior to Miranda, he said. So, an active sexual relationship was a welcome, intoxicating lifestyle change. They often came together in that way (pun intended).

So, when Peter's interest began to wane, and when his physical response to her began lessening, Miranda noticed right away.

*What's happening?* she worried.

○

Peter grew up in an environment much like mine, with small-town, Christian values, and like me, he had an authentic desire to be a good man whom people liked and respected. A good man like his father. Everyone liked his dad. Everyone seemed to think his dad was a good guy. So, young Peter learned that acting like his father resulted in people liking you and being nice to you.

*Good boy.*

But Peter's dad had secrets.

Alcoholism, for one. And a propensity for corporal punishment, for another. Sometimes, if Peter's mom told his dad that Peter had been misbehaving that day, his dad would escort young Peter to the basement and make him pull down his pants and underwear and put both of his hands on the wall. Maybe he said something like *"Why do you make me do this, Peter?"* or *"You know, this is going to hurt me more than it hurts you."*

Then, his dad would paddle him with a wooden cricket bat.

*Bad boy.*

This went on for several years until his dad eventually got sober and joined a church community.

With his dad no longer hitting him, young Peter's fear of his father lessened, and he wanted to spend more time with him. Sometimes he would seek out his father working in the family barn, hoping to help out and learn new skills. But Dad would always shoo him away.

As an early teen, Peter one day ventured into the barn when his dad wasn't home. He climbed a ladder to the barn's loft where he'd been warned to never go. And that's where he discovered a secret room.

There were countless adult magazines and pornographic videos in a makeshift living room with a chair and a television. Peter didn't know this room existed and didn't believe anyone besides his father knew it was there either. Peter had never seen images like the ones in the magazines and on the video covers.

Busty, sultry, naked women. They didn't look like the girls at school. They didn't look like his mother or sisters, all of whom were petite with brown hair.

*So, this is what Dad is really doing when he's out here. He's not working. He's looking at naked women.*

Peter returned the pornography stash to how he had found it. He ran back to the house, unable to tell anyone about what he had found because he wasn't supposed to be there.

*Bad boy.*

○

I'm not a psychiatrist or psychologist. But it seems that my coaching client Peter developed two key beliefs as a young boy that would later yield severe consequences for Miranda and his marriage.

The first belief Peter developed was the idea that you were supposed to marry women who looked and acted like his mother and sisters. Conservative clothing and behavior. Nary a whisper of anything sexual or what anyone in town or in school or at church might consider to be indecent.

But that's not the kind of woman Peter met and fell in love with. *Miranda is the kind of woman you want to touch. Miranda is the kind of woman you fantasize about going to bed with. But Miranda is not the kind of woman with whom you settle down and have kids. Miranda is not someone who will fit in at family dinners and holiday get-togethers,* Peter thought.

The second belief Peter developed that would later do harm to his marriage is that it's perfectly normal and okay to be married with children, do and say things that result in friends and neighbors thinking and feeling that you're a good man, and have a secret life steeped in sexual fantasy outside of marriage.

Peter's secret fantasies didn't necessarily involve busty, sultry, naked women. He already had one of those.

Peter's secret fantasies involved old high school crushes. Soccer moms he might meet at Little League games where he was coaching his kids. Co-workers. Women he dated before marriage.

He'd look them up on Facebook. And he'd "like" their photos. Sometimes he would send them messages under the guise of neighborly friendship. Other times, they read as something less veiled, like the time he sent a recently divorced woman who happened to be an old high school crush a message offering a shoulder to cry on while they commiserated about their tattered relationships.

Peter and Miranda's marriage was indeed tattered. Sex was less intimate, less satisfying, and less often. Questions about why were met with avoidance. With defensiveness. With invalidation.

Miranda didn't understand why any of this was happening. She was scared. *Maybe he doesn't love me. Maybe he doesn't want me. Maybe there's someone else,* she thought. *But that CAN'T be. Peter is such a shy,*

*reserved, conservative guy. That would be so out of character for him. He's
not capable of that.*

She didn't understand why Peter's father acted so strangely around
her or why her father-in-law made her feel uncomfortable. Miranda
tried to fit in with Peter's family but felt little but coldness and rejection
from his mother and sisters.

When his wife relayed these feelings to Peter, he dismissed her concerns as paranoia. He accused her of bad-mouthing his family and he
defended their behavior.

And then she discovered his secret Facebook habits. The pieces of
the puzzle started falling into place.

Ironically, Peter could have had the most rabid porn habit on planet
Earth, and if he'd only been transparent with Miranda about it, they
would have gotten along just fine.

Miranda wasn't hurt because Peter had private fantasies.

Miranda was hurt because Peter, it turned out, WAS capable of
things she had never considered possible. The truth hit hard and painfully: For a decade, wool had been pulled over her eyes. She had no
idea who her husband really was or what he was capable of.

On that day, Miranda's world ended.

Peter never set out to hurt anyone. Certainly not his wife and children. But because he chose secrecy (and never questioned whether
it was okay because good, married men have secret sexual fantasies
and habits, he had learned at a young age) and because he took his
family's side against his wife's, whatever trust Miranda had for Peter
vanished.

Miranda's storybook marriage had become a nightmare. Zero trust.
Zero safety.

And now Peter was facing the possibility of losing his wife and children. Like me, life was painfully, mercilessly making Peter feel the consequences of his choices.

He never set out to hurt anyone. He would have done everything differently had he known then what he knows now. He may be an exceptionally good guy. He seems that way when you talk to him.

But a broken wife and family are the fruits of his adult choices.

○

My wife never really knew who I was sexually. I was always too shy or too afraid to talk about it.

So, in some ways, we spent years with our marriage never really having a chance because I was too chicken-shit to discuss real things with her.

When two people promise to never have sex with anyone else again, it stands to reason that—unless you despise orgasms or physical intimacy or prefer sexual repression—you and your partner must make your bedroom (or wherever!) experiences good to avoid either of you craving something more or different in ways that might ultimately destroy your relationship.

This can't be repeated enough: **When we are obstacles to our partner's individual pursuits of happiness—their climb up the human-needs ladder or pyramid—then we are complicit in their eventual decision to choose a life in which the person who promised to love them forever isn't, at best, negligently holding them back.**

That's not to imply that infidelity is sometimes justified. I can think of no situation in which betraying another's trust seems like the right thing to do—particularly someone with whom we might share homes and children and to whom we promised the rest of our lives.

I do not believe there's some virtuous argument to be found for betraying one's spouse. But can I understand why someone in a relationship who has for many years felt unloved, unappreciated, undesired, neglected, and perhaps abused might succumb to the advances of an attractive someone else who treated them well?

Of course. I totally get that. Cause and effect.

This doesn't mean that victims of infidelity should be blamed for their partner's transgressions. That would be gross. But I think it means that we should accept the great responsibility of treating our partners in ways, and behaving in ways, that result in them WANTING to be with us and no one else.

We achieve trust in our relationships when we behave in ways that mathematically result in trust formation. We generate trust by being honest, consistent, and vulnerable.

I was dishonest with my wife about sex-related things in our marriage. I was, in general, uncomfortable discussing sex audibly in conversation. But I was mostly afraid of disclosing everything that I thought and felt and feared and fantasized and wanted or didn't want.

Why?

It's a messy combination of things, some fear-based, and some nobly intended, but still bullshitty and relationship damaging.

**The first reason** is that I was trying to fit myself into the This Is How a Husband Is Supposed to Think of His Wife box. Not everyone will be able to relate to that. So, let's back up for a minute to my formative years to give you an idea of what kind of box we're talking about.

I grew up in a small Ohio town in middle America. About 20,000 residents. Surrounded for many miles by even smaller rural communities. I come from a Christian family. A Catholic one. And, in my childhood home, a great emphasis was placed on practicing our faith. It's common to meet Catholics who don't follow every church teaching to the letter. You might call them casual practitioners of Catholicism. We were no such family.

I attended Catholic school from first grade through high school graduation. We never missed Sunday mass, even if we were out of town for road trips or vacations.

I was taught that it is impolite to discuss religion and politics at the dinner table, but the two were pervasive and intertwined in our home. Jesus was our copilot, and he wanted us to avoid sin so that we could go to heaven after we die, and he wanted us to vote Republican every two to four years while we were waiting to go there.

*"Hey, Matt! This is interesting and all, but I'm neither Christian nor particularly conservative. What the hell does this have to do with me and my life?"*

People may quibble philosophically with the notion that places like the United States and many countries throughout the world are Christian nations, but the math is pretty convincing. No matter your spiritual beliefs, Christianity's reach and impact has been enormous through the centuries and likely affects your life in ways you might not have considered.

While only 33 percent of people globally identify themselves as Christians, the vast majority of the English-speaking world (the only language in which I can speak and write fluently) identifies as Christian. That's 83 percent of Americans, 76 percent of Europeans, 80 percent of South Africans, and about half of the populations of Australia and New Zealand.

I wouldn't dream of trying to speak for other Christians, Catholics, or even the other kids I grew up with. I don't pretend to know what they thought and felt back in school.

I only know what I thought and felt, but what adulthood has taught me is that when you think and feel something, you tend to discover that millions of other people think and feel those things too.

It is safe to say that the common Christian teaching around sex might be negatively affecting young people in ways that has produced generations of people who hide their sexual desires or activities out of shame, which then later leads to relationship-destroying trust issues in marriage.

**Note:** I am NOT saying that I believe Christianity or conservative religious life of any kind is somehow bad. I would never. In fact, I can't think of one time in more than forty years that I heard of a relationship ending because two people positioned their faith as the central and most sacred thing in their lives. Faith and membership in a church community provide foundational stability for individuals and families. Something on which to anchor rather than drift aimlessly through life. That steadiness helps a lot of people. It helped me. For whatever I may believe today, I have only gratitude and positive things to report about my upbringing. What we lacked in financial resources in my youth was more than made up for in family and friends. We were—I was— abundantly blessed.

I don't think religion or faith is somehow the problem. But I do believe that teaching religion in the way I was taught might be ac- cidentally creating a human condition that fundamentally harms marriages and, by proxy, families. (And I have never met a religious person, teacher, or leader who wanted to harm marriage.)

This accidental damage resulting from the way some young people are taught about religion commonly leads to several marriage-killing conditions, including:

- Secret pornography use.

- Sexual anxiety that can adversely affect intimacy and performance, resulting in one or both spouses not wanting to do it for fear it will go poorly.

- Discomfort discussing sex, which can prevent intimacy building and lead to spouses questioning our own desirability and self-worth.

- A belief that all sexual thoughts and desires and activities are sinful and taboo outside of marriage, which can create a psychological condition where forbidden sex becomes a turn-on in a way "approved" sex with one's spouse never could. The negative implications of which should be obvious. The concept of forbidden fruit is the central plot device in the Christian Bible's human origin story.

Here were my takeaways from the few teachings on masturbation handed down to me as a young person in Catholic school. Even if this doesn't sound like anything you've ever thought or felt, I encourage you to consider whether you have ever dated or married (or might in the future) someone operating on a similar belief system.

1. My friends and I were taught growing up that any sexual thoughts we had or actions we took were sinful (if we weren't married, and none of us were because we were little kids).

I don't mean sinful like *"That's naughty!"*

I mean sinful like *"If you die—which could literally happen any minute—Jesus is going to be so disappointed in you that he might send you to hell for eternity!"*

Have you guys ever spent a couple of hours in a hospital waiting room? Stood in line at the DMV? Got stuck in a traffic jam when you were in a huge hurry? That's just hours. Eternity is FOREVERRRRR-RRRRRRRRRRRRRRRRR.

I basically imagine eternal damnation as the shittiest time in your life you can possibly think of. The worst you have ever felt. So maybe it's a few weeks after your divorce, and your ex is dating someone else who probably has a PhD and a ten-inch penis, and you're crying a lot and afraid of everything because you're going to die alone. And then one day you're, like, working it out in the shower or wherever drenched in loneliness and shame, and it turns out that everyone else in the world is watching you do this because you're secretly the star of a real-life, hidden-camera *The Truman Show,* and then out of nowhere someone randomly emails you the video that the rest of the world just watched along with a chiding note: *"Everyone knows, loser!!! Even your mom and grandma!!!"* And then you peek nervously out the side window of your house and there's your seventy-year-old neighbor lady pointing and laughing at you too. And then, because you're in hell for jerking it like a crying, lonely loser, God is going to banish you there for eternity so that you can feel that exact feeling every day, forever. Not for two weeks. Not for a thousand years. You're going to be stuck in that shit show forever and ever. Permanently. A special kind of torture without end.

I'm not saying that's what adults were TRYING to convey to us. But that's what was conveyed to us. At least to me. And you know what? Maybe it's true. Maybe there is some special place in hell for crying divorcées who masturbate. I don't have any way of knowing. What I know is that your marriage can get really unpleasant when you believe all of those things and combine it with the following.

2. *Masturbation is weird and gross!* I'd think. *I can't talk about that! Only losers and virgins do that! You can tell because the other kids at school are always making jokes about it! I guess there's something wrong with me. There's no chance any of the adults in church would ever do something like that! Why would they when they're all happily married and regularly having sex with their spouses?!*

Practicing Catholics go to confession periodically if not regularly. Inside the confessional, one has a private conversation with a priest, confessing their sins or disclosing things they are feeling guilty about. The idea is that God forgives you via the priest's intercession.

Even though I'm a dreadful Catholic by the standards of my upbringing, I've been to confession in adulthood. One time when I was still married, I was in the confessional and I mentioned this whole masturbation thing. The priest could tell I was nervous and uncomfortable discussing it.

"How often?" he asked. I told him. His reply: "That's it?! You're not even trying!"

Hilarious as it was, the chasm between his implied permission and my childhood beliefs that all masturbators will endure an eternity of fiery torment is pretty wide.

3. My final takeaway from childhood religious education regarding masturbation: once puberty hit, allowing all of the sexy-time energy to pile up for weeks, months, and years didn't seem plausibly sustainable.

I don't imagine that most young people growing up in religious households sit around thinking *"Gee willikers! What should I do to entertain myself right now? Oh, I know! Diddle my privates!"*

I imagine it's more along the lines of "*Good God, man. I really need to do it with someone, because holy shit. But unfortunately I'm only like 14 years old and don't know how. Besides, we are supposed to wait for marriage because premarital sex is a sin too! And premarital sex seems like an even-BIGGER sin than this private, by-myself sin. So, I guess I'll just watch this weird scrambled adult TV channel that is mostly snowy static, because I can totally see a naked boob once in a while.*" Or, you know, whatever.

**The second reason** I wasn't fully honest and transparent with my wife about sex is because I was afraid of her judgment and rejection. I don't mean to imply that she was an overly judgmental person to me or anyone else. I was probably projecting my mountain of insecurities onto her without giving her a fair chance to deal with them honestly.

Because I had so much pent-up fear and shame about sex, I associated my sexual fantasies with the notion of being bad. Not in the fun, naughty way. Actual bad-bad. And it felt wrong to imagine my wife—this woman I loved and honored and felt protective of—within the framework of all of this poisonous lusty wrongness.

I was afraid of her knowing about my sexual appetites because I was afraid she'd see me as some unlovable deviant to whom she wouldn't want to be married.

I never gave her the chance of accepting or rejecting the most honest, unmasked version of me because I was a scared kid and prioritized my wants and comforts over her short- and long-term well-being, though at the time, I didn't know how to think about it that way.

**The third reason** I hid things from my wife was the only noble one—I didn't want to hurt her feelings. She's a lovely woman. Beautiful. Seriously. It wasn't her fault that she couldn't magically transform into spicy Asian triplets or a large-breasted brunette covered in sexy tattoos and body piercings. I'm not the type of guy who ogles women publicly or would tell my wife how attractive I thought some celebrity on television was. I never wanted to communicate anything that could be interpreted as me believing she wasn't good enough, even though I ended up doing that anyway all while acting as if she were the one with the problem.

**The fourth reason** is that I honestly believed I would outgrow these thoughts and feelings. You sit around being seventeen or twenty-four or thirty-two, and you keep thinking *I wonder when I'm going to stop having all of these thoughts and feelings like the adults who always seem as if they have it all together!* It isn't until much later that we learn that personal growth is a choice and that all of those adults we believed had mastered life also have their own private battles, insecurities, fears, failures, and feelings of weakness. People always do. We just didn't know about it, because this is neither polite nor comfortable dinner-table conversation.

We grow up comparing ourselves to an imaginary standard we apply to the adults we know and are constantly falling short without realizing that the adults feel more or less the same way that we do.

We walk around feeling like we're the only ones in the world who think and feel these things. And it's lonely, especially in those quiet moments when we're alone with our thoughts. Lying in bed. Staring at the ceiling. Wondering *What's wrong with me?*

Everything? Nothing? You're a person, just like me. Just like my ex-wife. Just like Peter. Just like Miranda.

Whatever it is that you think and feel but have maybe always been too afraid to say out loud to anyone—you're not the only one.

## SEXUAL BELIEFS AND BEHAVIOR IN RELATIONSHIPS HAVE A PROFOUND EFFECT ON TRUST

Nicole fell in love with Ben and accepted his invitation to move in with him. *"He's the one,"* she thought.

The young couple settled into the ebb and flow of cohabitation, which introduces us to life similarly to how we will experience it in marriage. Shared expenses. Shared meals. Shared chores. Shared plans. And a shared bed.

One time, after several months of living together, Nicole hopped onto Ben's laptop computer to perform a task, and—BAM—she found an adult entertainment advertisement for casual sex encounters.

She was devastated. *"Oh my God. He's meeting strangers for cheap sex! I can't believe how stupid I am! How did I not realize this?"*

Ben was not who she believed him to be, she decided. Nicole felt as if she couldn't trust herself. She felt rejected and disgusted. She felt betrayed.

Nicole, experiencing betrayal trauma, confronted Ben with the discovery. He laughed once he realized what was happening.

"It's not what you think, babe."

It turned out that what Nicole had discovered wasn't Ben trying to hook up with local strangers but instead was a random pop-up ad, which isn't uncommon when visiting pornographic websites, not that I would know anything about that, Mom.

Ben had been looking at porn. Which for some couples is trust-breaking enough to end a relationship. I don't know whether porn was a major breach of trust for Nicole. The main reason I like this story so much is because it illustrates how much damage can be caused in the absence of transparency.

You get to think whatever you want about pornography in terms of its level of harmfulness. We'll talk more about that in a bit. But, if we're playing the relativism game, I'm guilty of believing that looking at internet porn is a more palatable activity than secretly cheating on your live-in girlfriend with strangers.

The last time I was inside of a strip club, I was twenty-three years old and had recently relocated from Ohio to Florida following college graduation. After attending a Major League Baseball spring training game, my buddy and I decided to hit a strip club for drinks at the Cheetah Lounge in Sarasota, Florida. My girlfriend—my future ex-wife—had moved to Florida too, though we had not yet moved in together.

A couple of the Cheetah dancers came to our table and sat down with us. My friend and I were politely flirting with them as the twenty-three-year-old versions of us were wont to do.

After leaving the club and heading home, I discovered that I'd accidentally pocket-dialed my girlfriend from the strip club earlier. She was upset because she'd heard me being friendly with another woman.

Knowing I'd done nothing inappropriate (minus the lack of transparency) I laughed at my crying girlfriend—but not in a mocking way. I honestly thought it was funny that she didn't understand. Every guy—at least every guy with as little money as I had—knew that the LAST place to meet women authentically interested in you or who you might hook up with—was a strip club. And so, when I realized she was upset because she thought I was legitimately flirting with other girls at a bar, I thought the fact that I was at a strip club and behaving as gentlemanly as one can in that environment, was actually a super-valid defense.

It was easy for me to dismiss my girlfriend's anxiety and pain because of how ludicrous I considered it to imagine me legitimately trying to connect with a young strip club employee. (The empathy lessons I've learned since my divorce would have served me well then.)

Ben's story about the porn website pop-up ads felt to me much like this experience, which I told him about during our first coaching call.

Here's the part that is really important. Do you remember the hypothetical morgue prank from Chapter 5? Where you maybe spent untold minutes or hours truly believing that your friend or family member had died? Feeling all of those shocked and grieving feelings?

Well, it was the same for the woman who would eventually give birth to our son when she believed she was hearing direct evidence that she didn't mean as much to me as she thought.

And it was the same for Nicole.

Regardless of what Ben was doing or not doing, there was a moment in which Nicole literally experienced betrayal trauma because she was convinced that he was using the internet to meet other women.

Even if we as parents know there is no monster hiding under the bed, sometimes our kids—legitimately, in their very real lived experience—are terrified.

Even if Ben believes—similarly to what I believed during the strip-club incident—that the basis for Nicole's fear and anxiety was dismissible based on the fact that he didn't do what she feared most, Nicole was still mentally and emotionally experiencing life as if he had.

We can debate whether this is fair. Feel however you'd like about your level of responsibility for other people's emotions. But if you're interested in being part of a peaceful, healthy, sustainable, long-term romantic relationship or marriage, then I would encourage you to value—intensely—the level of trust between you and your partner. It doesn't matter that you're not out there sticking your privates inside of other people's privates. If your partner has authentic fear and anxiety related to betrayals either with you or from a past relationship, then I beg you to show up for her or him in a way that communicates how much their well-being matters to you.

○

So, I didn't talk to my wife openly and honestly about sex. I don't want to blame Jesus, my parents, or my Catholic upbringing for my failed marriage. We are all responsible for our choices. But that whole bit about fearing masturbatory and premarital sex hellfire is seriously the reason all the sex stuff got weird with me. I had a lot of fear and shame related to beliefs about sex that turned out to be an unhealthy handicap in the context of marriage.

One of the most common stories you hear about situations like this involves the guy who sneaks off with his phone or to the computer late at night or when no one else is home to look at porn photos or watch videos.

I've never been a rampant porn consumer and I swear I'm not just saying that. Real people just always seemed hotter to me than "fake" people in photos or videos.

But I've still been the guy whose wife turned on the shared home computer to find some minimized pop-up web page full of porn images a few times.

I realize there are many people unfazed by pornography consumption, whether it be their own use or their romantic partner's.

But I also know that many do care. They are fazed. And for those who care, trust is at stake—the marriage ingredient that we need most.

Some people don't like their partner consuming porn because it results in them feeling insecure, as if they are not attractive enough or good enough to pleasure their partners and satisfy them sexually. Some people consume porn because their sex lives are inconsistent or nonexistent, and I think about some guy's wife wrestling with a bunch of uncomfortable questions about why he doesn't seem sexually interested in her when they're going weeks or months without physical intimacy.

And then she discovers he's watching porn.

And she's like *"Wait a fucking minute. I totally want to have sex with you, even though you're a shitty husband half the time. I have actual, physical, touchable body parts with a working vagina and everything, and you're sneaking around getting off to airbrushed, fake-breasted electronic chicks on a screen with your dick in your hand?!"*

So, guys. Mental exercise: Think of your best guy friend. Or one of your partner's platonic guy friends. Maybe a co-worker. And now, imagine your wife has rejected your sexual advances for several weeks and you're starting to worry about it and wonder why.

And then one day you come home to find her masturbating while looking at a picture of your friend or some other guy she knows while moaning his name. Super into it too.

Can you picture it?

That might be close to how she feels when she realizes you never touch her or tell her she's sexy or beautiful or that you want her but that you're wanking it to internet chicks.

Just maybe, if you don't wank it to internet chicks and you DO tell her that she's sexy and beautiful (and perhaps more substantial observations about what makes her a desirable and admirable and interesting person) a bunch of really positive neato things will begin to manifest between the two of you. Worth a try?

## THE SEXUAL MOTIVATION PROBLEM

One of my favorite writers, Mark Manson, in his book *Models: Attract Women Through Honesty* tackled the subject of porn and masturbation in dating without filtering it through the prism of religion or morality.

This applies to modern marriage too.

Part of making your marriage awesome involves behaving in ways that result in your spouse feeling respected, safe, loved, desired, and sexy so that you can have a kick-ass and bond-forming sex life together. When you stop pursuing your spouse emotionally and sexually as you did when you were dating, it can result in them feeling less loved, less desired, and less sexy and, thusly, feeling less safe in the relationship.

And even though that's true, she or he may still want to have sex with you a lot. When you're getting off by yourself all the time, you eliminate your physical and psychological motivation to pursue your partner.

Manson wrote *"There's a bit of an epidemic of sexual apathy going on worldwide, where husbands, boyfriends, and even single men are turning to pornography rather than the real life women that they see walking around every day. And it makes sense why: it's easier . . . the sex is more exciting, it's available at any time . . . the girls never say no, and . . . there are no obligations or commitments involved.*

*"The problem is that there are some negative side effects. The first being that porn creates very, very unrealistic expectations about sex, about women, and about sexuality. Porn makes money by accentuating and exaggerating sexual ideals. Actual sex with an actual woman often involves awkward moments of figuring out what she likes, what you like,*

*who likes it which way. It also involves ecstatic moments of emotional intimacy, something porn can never provide . . .*

*"The other problem is that porn is so easy, that it encourages men to masturbate . . . a lot. And as we all know, as men, the more we masturbate, the more interested we become in food and television, and the less we become in women and accomplishing something . . .*

*"Science is starting to back this up. Orgasms, or more accurately, ejaculation in men, actually causes a depletion of various hormones and endorphins which often lead to useful behaviors as well as motivation."*

○

You probably already know this, but you will get bored with pretty much everything in your life.

I classify it as hedonic adaptation, but maybe it is something else.

It is an important concept to understand because when people don't know what we are up against, we are more likely to experience hardship and failure.

Hedonic adaptation is the psychological phenomenon of our brains adjusting to positive (or negative) life changes and normalizing them, which results in our brains and bodies returning to their baseline happiness levels once we've adapted to the life change. The consequences of this include losing some of the emotional highs (or lows) we used to feel upon first experiencing them.

For example, let's pretend you get a new job with a significant pay raise. It feels good. You feel richer. But then you get used to it. Your brain adapts to your new income level. And then maybe you feel more or less the same as you did before.

I've gotten four new jobs since earning my university diploma, each pay increase more significant than the last. But I never felt richer than when I went from a poor, just-scraping-by college student to my whopping $28,000 per year salary as a young, inexperienced newspaper reporter in 2002.

Another good example is getting a new car. It feels good climbing into it or seeing it parked outside of your house or sitting in your garage. You're really proud of it. You handpick individual pet hairs and pieces of rock or dirt from the carpet to keep it clean. But as time goes on, you get used to the new car. Then, if you're like me, you let it get just as dirty as your old car.

I don't know whether psychology experts will approve of me using hedonic adaptation for framing the human condition of lessening sexual attraction over time between two people, but it's the way that I think about it.

People are uncomfortable with the idea of comparing how we feel about "things" like money and cars to how we feel about the people we are supposed to love.

As a recovering idealist, I totally understand where they are coming from. It's an insult to the sacredness of marriage and the intrinsic value of a human being to reduce a person—and certainly a spouse—to an object.

But an idea being uncomfortable should not disqualify it from being true. I don't think our brains give a shit WHAT the thing/person/ experience is. I believe it's a foregone conclusion that as familiarity and comfort with something grows, the likelihood that you'll take it for granted through thoughtlessness increases.

I don't think it's a foregone conclusion that you will love or value someone or something less. Only that you are likely to forget in the busyness of daily life how much these people or things matter to you.

Not unlike our ability to breathe or see or have use of our arms and legs. People tend to take them for granted until the least fortunate among us loses one of these blessings.

It's not ideal. But it is the human condition.

Those chemical triggers that make young couples crush on one another and lust for one another when they first meet will, 100 percent, no exceptions, lose intensity or disappear entirely over time.

It's TOTALLY uncomfortable to suggest to your spouse or partner that you—in a base-mammal way—aren't as attracted to them as you once were. I think that's why most people avoid discussing it. We tend to avoid uncomfortable conversations and situations.

It turns out that one of the inconvenient truths about sexual attraction is the existence of a biological phenomenon observed in animals (including people) called the Coolidge Effect, which demonstrates that sexual interest increases or is renewed when a new partner is introduced to have sex with, even after stoppage of sex with a prior, but still available, partner.

This behavior can be observed with both genders, but researchers report seeing the Coolidge Effect in males at a higher rate than females (though I don't know whether that research factors in culturally induced gender roles like "slut shaming" and objectification or the sexual abuse females experience at a much higher rate than males).

The Coolidge Effect was named by behavioral endocrinologist Frank A. Beach in 1958, as documented in Roger N. Johnson's 1972 book *Aggression in Man and Animals*. Beach shared an old joke about US president Calvin Coolidge's marriage.

"The President and Mrs. Coolidge were being shown [separately] around an experimental government farm. When [Mrs. Coolidge] came to the chicken yard she noticed that a rooster was mating very frequently. She asked the attendant how often that happened and was told, 'Dozens of times each day.' Mrs. Coolidge said, 'Tell that to the President when he comes by.' Upon being told, the President asked, 'Same hen every time?' The reply was, 'Oh no, Mr. President, a different hen every time.' President: 'Tell that to Mrs. Coolidge.'"

Please don't read this as being some veiled advocacy for polyamory. I promise that it's not. Please live the life you want to live. The idea of sharing a romantic partner with other people is mentally, spiritually, and emotionally complicated, and I don't pretend to have any answers.

I've long believed that nearly any type of romantic relationship structure can work so long as the participants are philosophically aligned and both rowing their metaphorical boats in the same direction. Decide for yourself whether trust can exist between two people in an open relationship.

Instead of questioning whether marriage should or should not be structured as it is, it's more practical and pragmatic to accept simply that it is structured as it is.

About 95 percent of adults are married, were once married, or plan to marry. It's important that we keep in mind the influence the institution of marriage has on our lives and society, regardless of how any individual might feel about it.

I also believe it's intellectually dishonest to pretend as if two unmarried people in a long-term romantic relationship together don't more or less require the same level of trust and emotional connection with one another as they would in marriage to live peaceful, fulfilling lives.

o

Our ability to navigate intimate relationships effectively is of paramount importance to our quality of life.

Finding this peace and fulfillment will inevitably require getting a little uncomfortable and engaging in meaningful conversations with the people we care about to achieve trust and intimacy.

I don't know about you, but aside from the well-intentioned but mostly useless warning that *"Marriage is hard work!"* I was not armed in my youth with any of the emotional-intelligence tools and relationship skills I've worked hard to cultivate in my post-divorce adult life.

And I wonder *How much different might things have been had I entered my marriage with a legitimate understanding of what I needed to know in order to succeed?*

I know it hurts when you break up with someone. I know it hurts when people you like don't seem to like you back. I know it hurts when people seem to value a relationship less than you do. But I also know that no girlfriends, boyfriends, wives, husbands, friends, strangers, nor anyone else on earth gets to decide what you're worth. What she's worth. What he's worth. What I'm worth.

You do.

I do.

# 10

# WHAT MATTERS VS. WHAT DOESN'T

IN JUNE OF 2001, I WAS SPENDING MY LAST SUMMER SCHOOL BREAK living out of state at my dad and stepmom's house and working as an intern reporter for one of the local daily newspapers. This was just one academic calendar year shy of starting the rest of my life.

I was taking a summer Spanish language class at a local community college, and I was working on a homework assignment for that class when the house phone rang. (We were still several years away from pretty much everyone having their own mobile phone.) My dad answered it. "Yes, he's right here. Just a second." He held the phone out to me. "It's for you."

*"Hello?"*

She said hi, and my heart did a whole thing. It was a girl from my university back in Ohio. I hadn't talked to her or seen her in several months. Mutual friends had introduced us at a keg party about halfway through our freshman year. We talked a lot that first night. Dozens of others were there too, but I don't remember many of them. I drank a lot of beer that night because I used to be all about drinking a lot of beer. I got sick and puked in the party host's only bathroom.

Despite this very poor first showing, she had liked me anyway.

She was pretty. And I understand that attraction is a subjective experience, but she was the kind of pretty that hurts a little bit—something I rarely experienced outside of a particularly attractive AND likable movie or TV actress who makes you involuntarily crush on her (think Danica McKellar in *The Wonder Years* when you're a grade-school kid or Minka Kelly in *Friday Night Lights*). She was a dancer for the university's basketball team. Our school's equivalent of the Laker Girls. I remember sitting in the arena stands, elbowing my friends, like "Dude. Where the hell are these girls? Why don't we ever see them at parties?"

Turns out, while my crew was drinking excessively and smoking copious amounts of marijuana, these young ladies were busy working out, practicing choreography, and actually applying themselves to academic study—a habit and lifestyle that didn't particularly interest me at the time. (Sorry, Dad.)

In addition to all of the achingly attractive on-court dancing she was doing with her too-busy-for-parties troupe, she was also the feature baton twirler for the university marching band.

I enjoyed going to football and basketball games because I really like football and basketball. But for the following four years, she was always at those games, front and center, shining brightly, taking me back to that night I'd met her over cheap keg beer at my friend Scott's dining room table. I imagine most people watch all of the pretty dancing girls when they run out to the court for time-outs and halftime shows. I imagine most people's eyes dart around to all of the marching band members while they're doing their thing on the football field.

But I always watched her, specifically. Because, you know.

"I know that girl," I'd say to anyone who would listen in a way that I hoped seemed non-braggy, even though I was totally bragging. "She's awesome. We almost had a thing freshman year, and still talk periodically."

She and I had a running joke for the entirety of 1999 that if any of the Y2K doomsday scenarios played out when the calendar flipped to January 1, 2000, we were going to find each other and bunker down in the apocalypse together. Anytime I'd talk to her after that, I'd always half-jokingly feign disappointment that the world hadn't ended, lamenting the lost opportunity to be with her.

And so, standing behind the bar in my father's basement, twenty-two years old, all sorts of feelings bubbled up hearing her voice on the phone—someone I didn't necessarily think I would ever see again.

She had somehow tracked down my dad's phone number. Five hundred miles away. Many months after our last conversation. Some of my friends must have helped her.

I told her it was great to hear from her and asked why she was calling. She had earned her diploma the previous spring and was preparing to move from Ohio to Orlando, Florida, with a couple of her girlfriends to start a new life.

That's awesome, I said. I told her that I was planning to move to Florida, too, after graduation because Florida was one of the best places to practice newspaper journalism. Lots of crazy news. Lots of competition. And, being from the occasionally snowy and cloudy Midwest,

I was supremely interested in living somewhere with palm trees and sandy beaches.

This was it. She was just days away from moving down there, but she was dealing with a nagging voice in her head, she said. A what-might-have-been whisper she had been hearing about me.

I was moved. Flattered. Smitten. This could have been the plot for one of those romantic comedies that I might pretend to not like in an effort to appear more manly than I actually sometimes feel.

"*I was hoping to see you again before I moved away,*" she said. "*I need to know.*"

I took down her number and told her I'd call her back. The only way this was going to work was if my dad were willing to allow a young woman whom he had never met to fly into town and stay with us for a few days.

I went upstairs and found him in the kitchen.

"Dad. I need to ask you something."

## THE SECRET TO LONG-TERM COMPATIBILITY IN DATING AND MARRIAGE ISN'T HOW ALIKE WE ARE

COM·PAT·I·BIL·I·TY—*noun—1. a state in which two things are able to exist or occur together without problem or conflict 2. a feeling of sympathy and friendship; like-mindedness*

There are two kinds of compatibility, and I am under the impression that when the average person speaks about romantic compatibility, they are focusing on the No. 2 definition. Friendship. Like-mindedness. Similar personalities, interests, wants, life goals, etc.

The focus, to a certain extent, is on ALIKENESS or SAMENESS.

Which isn't without merit and helps to make a compelling argument for using romantic compatibility charts (as one might find in personality type assessments like the Myers-Briggs Type Indicator [MBTI] or the Enneagram of Personality) and other matchmaking tests.

I'm guilty of believing that a brothel-owning cocaine enthusiast and an Evangelical Christian are probably a bad match for long-term dating and marriage. I'm equally suspicious of a twenty-four-year-old hip-hop DJ in Brooklyn, New York, pursuing romance with a forty-seven-year-old botany professor in rural Oklahoma.

An argument can be made for being discriminatory in dating so that we are set up for success in a long-term relationship we enter.

*"What kind of dog should I get?"* I typed into Google one day.

Several sites popped up with dog breed selector tools and quizzes designed to help people find dogs best suited for their individual preferences, lifestyles, and living environments.

The American Kennel Club (AKC) makes its recommendations based on the following categories:

- Living Environment (House or Apartment)
- Number of Children
- Number of Other Dogs
- Typical Activity (at Home, Walking in Neighborhood, Going on Adventures)
- Noise Tolerance
- Cleanliness Preferences

Depending on your answers, the AKC returns a short list of recommended matches, almost like an eharmony for prospective pet owners.

*Why? How? Are the people at the American Kennel Club dog psychics?!*

Nope. They simply have decades, perhaps more than a century, of historical data that tells us that a puggle, an Old English sheepdog, and a Yorkshire terrier all will exhibit certain characteristics common to those particular breeds, just as a Siberian husky, French bulldog, and cocker spaniel will typically exhibit a different set of characteristics.

I believe this is a positive, useful, helpful practice. The results of successfully matching certain dog breeds with certain owner preferences are happy, healthy dogs delighting happy pet owners who generally aren't unpleasantly surprised by breed-specific behaviors.

Successfully matching certain dog breeds with owner preferences significantly reduces the amount of dogs being abandoned at shelters or by the side of the road, reducing demands on animal shelters and minimizing instances of euthanizing abandoned or stray pets in overpopulated shelters.

*"Hey, Matt! Why are you writing about dogs?! Have you been watching Space Buddies? What's your favorite dog breed? Pugs? Mastiffs? Are you super into Yorkies now?!"*

No. I'm not suddenly super into Yorkies.

After years of coaching and talking relationships every day, I'm super into the idea of being discriminating in dating and the partner selection processes to eliminate potential partners who are metaphorically liable to routinely shit on our floors and destroy our shoes. (Please note that I don't mean anything gross like racial discrimination. I mean that we should have more stringent, healthy filters prior to committed relationships to help combat the miserable-relationship epidemic.)

○

How well do you know your spouse or romantic partner? Your parents? Siblings? Best friends? If you took a personality test, answering questions how you imagine they would, how confident are you that the results would be accurate?

One of my former coaching clients had known and dated her fiancé for more than ten years and was three days away from her wedding the last time I spoke with her.

I ask many of my married or dating clients to take an online personality test rooted in the MBTI personality types. In MBTI, there are sixteen different personality types, and they are indicated by four letters. As mentioned previously, I am ENFP.

The first letter in MBTI can be either an E (extraversion) or an I (introversion).

The second letter is either an S (sensing) or an N (intuition).

The third letter is either a T (thinking) or an F (feeling).

And the fourth and final letter is either a J (judging) or a P (perceiving).

The Myers-Briggs personality test is a self-report inventory designed to identify someone's personality type, strengths, and preferences. The questionnaire was developed by Isabel Myers and her mother Katharine Briggs based on their work with Carl Jung's theory of personality types. Today, the MBTI inventory is one of the most widely used psychological instruments in the world, though it has been criticized by some scholars as a pseudoscience with the same scientific validity as astrology or fortune cookies. I care less about whether a particular method of measuring personality is scientifically valid and more about people getting intentional about knowing themselves and their partners for the purposes of optimized matchmaking.

Let the record show that, according to NASA astrophysicists, about 68 percent of the universe is comprised of dark energy (which we know literally nothing about other than the fact that we don't know anything about it) and another 27 percent of the universe is made up of dark matter (which scientists know how to detect with gravitational lensing but still know little to nothing about its actual composition). I'm no math genius, but that leaves us with only 5 percent of all observable "stuff" being identifiable, classifiable matter as you and I learned about it in school. Everything we can see, touch, and taste. Just 5 percent.

The smartest people on earth can't tell us what 95 percent of the universe's observable components are made of. They don't know. Soooo, if you sometimes subscribe to playfully illogical straw-man arguments like I do, maybe scientists who consider personality type study to be a waste of time can piss off. I don't pretend to know anything for sure. I just ask a lot of questions and mostly try to not be a dick to others with varying degrees of success.

There are a couple of reasons to ask people to take personality tests. The first is that self-knowledge is important. People don't always know themselves as well as they might think. And knowing ourselves can keep us away from all sorts of danger and out of toxic relationships. The second reason is because I often ask the people I coach to take the personality test an additional time but, that second time, answering the questions as they believe their partner would.

I love the insights and conversations that naturally occur when we discover the gaps between what we believe about someone else (or ourselves) and what's actually real. The majority of conflict that exists between two romantic partners lies in that gap between what we think we know and the truth.

So, I'm on the phone with this coaching client, Stacey, who is about to be married in a few days. And she's impressive. Brilliant. Master's degree holder. Objectively intelligent in measurable academic ways. And subjectively intelligent in all of the ways you experience when you're conversing with someone about life's big-picture stuff.

So, I was totally floored when I learned that Stacey got ALL FOUR LETTERS of her near-future husband's personality totally opposite when she took the test answering the questions as she believed he would.

When Stacey took the test, answering as she believed her fiancé, Chris, would, the results were INFP. But when Chris sent me the results of his own test, it was revealed that he is actually an ESTJ. It was a relationship coach's dream scenario. Not only did my brilliant client get her fiancé's personality traits 100 percent backward but it turns out that his personality profile is the same as hers.

Imagine what you're capable of believing about someone's intentions when you're filtering everything they do and say through an understanding of who they are that is 100 percent wrong.

We have got to get serious about not being so sure of ourselves all of the time. No matter how "smart" we are. We're wrong entirely too often to trust our own judgment as much as we do, and this affects both how we feel when things happen and how we treat other people.

Making a wise and disciplined partner selection in our romantic relationships begins with BEING someone a wise and disciplined partner would choose to be with. And hopefully we can be people who evaluate potential partners on the traits consistent with achieving durable, healthy relationships.

*Is this someone I can trust? Am I someone they can trust? Are we both willing to choose safety and trust over "being right" because we both—together and cooperatively—understand that we don't get to have a relationship without those conditions?*

# WHAT IF WE CREATE COMPATIBILITY?

**COM·PAT·I·BIL·I·TY**–*noun–a state in which two things are able to exist or occur together without problem or conflict*

It's natural to want to be with people who share our interests and values. And it's logical (although people somehow screw this up) to seek out a partner who has the same plans for having children and long-term family life.

But—and this is likely observably true in your own life—the interests and quirks and things people find attractive don't remain static. They change and evolve as we age and experience new things and new people.

Ted Hudson, a researcher at the University of Texas, conducted a longitudinal study on romantic compatibility in couples who had been married for several years.

*"My research shows that there is no difference in the objective compatibility between those couples who are unhappy and those who are happy,"* Hudson wrote.

Couples who feel content and positivity within their relationships said that compatibility wasn't an issue for them. The happy couples in Hudson's study said it was their own willful behavior that made the relationship successful—not personality compatibility.

When the unhappy couples in the study were asked about compatibility, they all said that compatibility was extremely important to having a successful marriage. And in the midst of their failing marriages, they didn't believe they were compatible with their partners.

When the unhappy couples said, *"We're incompatible,"* what they actually meant was *"We don't get along very well,"* Hudson wrote.

Therein lies the problem with the word "compatibility." Partners unhappy in their relationships often resort to blaming a lack of compatibility for their dysfunctional relationship.

Natural human chemistry brings people together romantically and sexually. We've been making babies and populating the planet using this method for longer than we've been recording history.

So, this is likely to keep happening.

Maybe someone who likes to go square dancing on the weekends can have an amazing relationship with an avid miniature golfer. Just maybe some competitive Pitmaster barbecue guy can have a beautiful family with a vegetarian spouse. After all, two people from the same town, who go to the same church and know all the same people and vote the same way and believe all the same things can have a colossally shitty marriage.

So maybe what we really need for compatibility with someone is about much more than our stated values. Maybe it's mostly about what we can actually demonstrate that we know and understand.

She wants to talk about it. It makes her feel better.

He doesn't want to talk about it. It makes him feel worse.

Are they incompatible?

Or.

Does being compatible really mean that she fundamentally understands how stressful and difficult conversations that may be cathartic for her can feel difficult and damaging for him, and then approaches conversations with him with that in mind?

And does being compatible really mean that he fundamentally understands that listening to what she has to say, even if it's inconvenient or a little bit frustrating for him, will strengthen the intimate bond between them, so he's going to make whatever concessions are necessary to achieve that?

Maybe being compatible means that two people are awake to the needs and wants of one another and that simple demonstrations of respecting and honoring those needs and wants—these little things many people never think about—create as a by-product all the feel-goodness that makes a person *feel* connected and compatible.

Love is a choice. Sure, it's a really damn hard choice after several years inside a shitty marriage, but it doesn't make it less true. Love is a choice.

Here's a quick five-step strategy for marriage success:

**STEP 1**–Know thyself.

**STEP 2**–Make a wise and disciplined partner selection.

**STEP 3**–If you want it to be for life, marry them.

**STEP 4**–Love them for who they are, not for what they do for you.

**STEP 5**–Repeat Step 4 every day forever.

## GETTING SERIOUS ABOUT OUR PERSONAL VALUES AND PERSONAL BOUNDARIES

It had been months since my pretty blonde friend from college had tracked me down at my dad's house from hundreds of miles away and hopped a plane to stay with us for a week and to accompany me as my date for my aunt's summer wedding.

She canceled her plans to move to Florida with her girlfriends to pursue a relationship with me. There was no turning back after that. This was storybook shit. And I had no regrets. Back in Ohio, fall classes were in session and we had settled into a boyfriend-girlfriend relationship in an apartment I rented alone near campus.

It was her first year in the workforce. My final year of college. My first year of not sharing an address with any roommates, though she visited frequently. We were dealing with the real-time emotional and psychological fallout from the September 11, 2001, terrorist attacks. And all of it felt like a big moment. It felt as if everything were about to change. I was wrapping up the classes and independent study projects I needed for my diploma and dreaming of moving to a Florida beach community to start my newspaper reporting career, where I assumed there would be nothing but the unending flow of ice-cold beer and umbrella drinks, along with a bunch of live reggae music surrounded by sun, surf, sand, and palm trees.

But there was trouble in paradise from jump street in that Ohio apartment before the Florida move happened. It turned out that my new girlfriend seemed much more emotionally volatile than I'd previously realized, and sometimes her ultrasensitive feelings were really cramping my style.

I was laid back. I didn't have fights. I didn't have conflict in my social relationships. People didn't get angry with me or criticize me or tell me how something I was doing was wrong.

Every experience I'd ever had with my family of origin, hometown friends, and the past few years of college taught me that I was likable and easy to get along with. I was the kind of person who woke up every day not only disinterested in harming others but never considering it. *I'm a good guy!*

So, when I started hearing about it from her when I'd agree to go to my friend's house for a Friday-night keg party (the most normal and routine of decisions throughout college) or because I'd grabbed dinner for myself without checking in with her first like she was my mother or something, I'd feel pretty pissed off and I wasn't afraid to say so.

"Ummm. Hey. I don't answer to you. I was hungry so I ate food. It's not as if we had made dinner plans." And also. "I'm not going to ask for permission to go to parties. These people are my best friends, and we're all about to graduate and maybe I won't see some of them very much for the rest of my life. You, on the other hand, I'm intending to move to Florida with to start a whole new life. Soooo, would you please chill out a bit? Because for the first time ever, I seriously want to spend the rest of my life with someone, and that someone is you."

I didn't understand that she was merely trying to feel seen and heard because, for her, a wise and disciplined partner selection involved being with someone who considered her needs and feelings when he made decisions and who didn't invalidate her pain when she expressed it.

I didn't understand that she only wanted to be considered when I was making dinner or social plans, because she knew that she needed to be someone I thought of as important enough to remember and think about when I was making decisions.

But as a twenty-two-year-old I was going to do what I wanted to do and I didn't want another person thinking they were going to be able to control me like a parent, or change me into someone I wasn't, no matter how great I thought she was. I was unwilling to compromise the autonomy I felt as a young adult (or big child) still finding my way in the world.

Eroding her trust—betraying it, really—began right away.

Sometimes she would cry. And not a discreet cry. An arms-hugging-the-knees, floor-sitting, body-rocking cry. Begging to be heard. Begging to be comforted. Begging to be loved.

And I didn't think that was okay. She was so hurt that her body wasn't doing all of the things she wanted it to do. And if I were in the frame of mind that it wasn't right for her to be upset about whatever she was upset about—I would respond emotionlessly. Cold. Uncaring. Not wanting to "reward" what I was considering to be unreasonable behavior with words or actions that communicated that I thought any of this was reasonable. Maybe I wasn't the good guy I believed myself to be.

From the start, I was capable of looking at this person I claimed to love experiencing real-time pain, and I did nothing to validate it, nothing to demonstrate empathy, nothing to communicate that what she felt mattered to me. I instead spent my energy trying to convince her that if she only thought thoughts and felt feelings more like the way I did, then she could stop feeling badly about these silly little things. I instead spent my energy defending myself and justifying my decisions.

*Why is she trying to make me responsible for her emotions?* I'd wonder. *This is absolute bullshit.*

o

What is a person worth? What are you worth? Who gets to decide?

Let's pretend I possess the world's largest diamond collection. Because diamonds have high market value, I would be "worth" a lot of money. But why are diamonds valuable? They're stones. Like the ones we skip across the surface of a lake and kick to the side of the hiking trail.

They're valuable because of supply-and-demand economics. When many people want something that isn't readily available, prices go up. The "value" goes up. It's why it is common to see empty seats at regular-season baseball and basketball games but you have to pay double or triple for standing-room-only tickets for playoff games. It's why price-gouging assholes on the internet could find buyers for hand sanitizer and disinfectant wipes during the outbreak of a global pandemic while most people couldn't find them in stock at their local stores.

Diamonds are rocks. They have a ton of market value as precious gemstones coveted by high-end jewelers and collectors. But they're just rocks. Just like paper money, treasury bonds, and gold coins, diamonds wouldn't be worth much in a postapocalyptic society following a global disaster.

Diamonds are useful for looking pretty (and cutting hard materials in manufacturing applications, but mostly just looking pretty).

Water, for example, is a much more useful substance than diamonds. Water provides life-sustaining support to plant and animal life. Our bodies are primarily composed of water. Water is fundamental and critical for sustaining biological life.

Without diamonds, everyone probably just buys ruby and emerald engagement rings. Without water, everything and everybody dies, and the planet turns into a desert wasteland.

Sometimes called the diamond-water paradox, diamonds and water best demonstrate the contradiction of water having much more usefulness and intrinsic value than diamonds, yet most of us dump water out on the ground or down drains every day.

Meanwhile, diamonds are among our highest-valued financial possessions. It's the paradox of value, a concept made famous by Scottish economist Adam Smith in the eighteenth century.

So, what do you think? What has greater value? Diamonds or water?

The idea of value—what a particular substance or item is worth—is purely subjective. In other words: **Each of us decides what we value, and then we spend our time and money accordingly.**

Can we agree that water is, in reality, much more valuable than diamonds? On account of one being predominantly for showing off your bling, while the other determines whether life will persist? I'm going to proceed as if we can.

But if the Diamond Fairy and Water Fairy both show up at my house today with a bucket of their finest offerings, I'm telling the Water Fairy to go kick rocks because of my functioning water faucets and bottled water readily available for purchase.

Of course, if I were dying of thirst in an ocean of desert sand, I'd make a different choice. It's a subjective experience.

It's not uncommon for someone feeling rejected while going through a breakup or suffering from the fallout of betrayal trauma to question their worth. One of my readers emailed me this question after a painful breakup: *"Please just tell me—am I worth something? I'm so lonely and sad. I ask myself, 'What is wrong with me that I'm not being valued?' It's so hard."*

I get it. When I realized what my wife was choosing over our marriage (namely sacrificing—very painfully—a ton of time with our son, among other social, family, and financial sacrifices) I too felt the full brunt of human rejection for the first time in my life.

The sky fell. My world ended.

And I truly understood what it looked and felt like to let other people influence how we feel about ourselves. *If she's willing to choose THAT, how much can I really be worth?*

I had a problem with this idea for most of my life.

If she liked some totally cliché and hokey romantic comedy better than some spectacularly awesome movie I liked, I would use some random metric to try to "prove" my preferences were more valuable than hers, like the number of positive movie reviews or a big box-office haul.

In this instance, it wasn't because I was trying to "win." I was trying to convince my wife to like the same things as me because I found it inconvenient that we often didn't like the same things, and I wanted to change that without me having to become an accomplished ballroom dancer or snow skier.

My strategy didn't work. People like different things and telling people that their opinions and preferences are "wrong" it turns out is unlikely to magically result in them changing their personal tastes.

But *why?*

There are four kinds of value. Maybe more. But at least these four:

1. **Intrinsic Value**—the idea of something having worth "in itself" or "in its own right."

   Human beings have intrinsic value. When we treat people as if they have intrinsic value, we don't murder, rape, rob, injure, defraud, defame, or otherwise harm them. Thus, it's a nice belief.

2. **Market Value**—a constantly fluctuating metric based primarily on supply and demand.

3. **Personal Value to Other People**

4. **Personal Value to Me**

So, what are you worth?

If you believe as most of us do, you have intrinsic value by virtue of being a living, breathing human being.

Your market value, however, depends entirely on context. If you are the world's best computer programmer, you're going to be the coolest and most "valuable" person in the room at your next conference or hackathon, but maybe you suck at other things, like long-distance swimming races or building a lumber deck or effectively training K-9 unit police dogs.

Your personal value to other people? I care about what others think of me even though it can get me into trouble. But when I get really intentional and thoughtful about this, I inevitably come to the conclusion that no one else's opinions matter. Some people eat cabbage and sauerkraut and canned spinach on purpose. Some people think chocolate tastes bad. Some people think ultra-tight skinny jeans look good on men. If disagreeing with them is wrong, I don't want to be right.

I can only conclude: **If the concept of value is purely subjective, then only an individual can determine her or his own worth, and others' opinions (or possibly just what we mistakenly believe they are) are unreliable and irrelevant data points in the equation.**

I know it hurts when you break up with someone. I know it hurts when people you like don't seem to like you back. I know it hurts when people seem to value a relationship less than you do. But I also know that no girlfriends, boyfriends, wives, husbands, friends, strangers, nor anyone nor anything else on earth gets to decide what you're worth. What she's worth. What he's worth. What I'm worth.

You do.

I do.

Diamonds or water? We decide. I can't tell you what to believe, but I can encourage you to decide for yourself that you matter, since your opinion is the only one that counts.

○

The words "values" and "boundaries" sounded like bullshit when I was growing up. They didn't sound like words that meant anything. They were just words adults used while droning on and on about things that didn't seem worth listening to.

When I was young, **I wasn't motivated to explore ideas like this or learn new things because everything was always good.** I was healthy and safe. I felt loved by family and accepted by friends. All of my needs were met. Because I never wanted for things, I never had to ask myself how to get something I wanted and then go through the growth process and hard work necessary to achieve it.

But then, just after I turned thirty-four, my wife left, and my son was no longer home every day. I was sad, angry, and ashamed. I was nothing like the happy and confident person I used to see in the mirror back when nothing was wrong. I was a broken, crying, terrified shell of that kid. *If I'm not that person anymore, who the hell am I?*

I didn't matter, and I knew it. I was weak, and I knew it. I wasn't worth a woman's love or desire, and I knew it.

Those were hard truths to accept, but life is really hard sometimes. After a lifetime of mostly blaming others when something went wrong because it was so much easier than accepting responsibility, I finally started asking the right questions:

*How did I get here? What could I have done differently to prevent this?*

The answer is simple enough: I didn't always live my values, and I didn't always enforce healthy boundaries.

What are values? **Your values are who YOU are, not who you think you should be to win the acceptance of others.**

"Values are the backbone of life," writes author Debra Smouse in a *Tiny Buddha* article. "If we don't know what's important to us, we spend a lot of time wandering and wondering what we should be doing. There is tremendous power in discovering and living according to our highest values and experiencing inner peace as the natural consequence."

What does it mean to enforce healthy boundaries? Having healthy boundaries means we take responsibility for our behavior and our feelings while NOT taking responsibility for others' behavior or emotions.

"People with poor boundaries typically come in two flavors: those who take too much responsibility for the emotions/actions of others, and those who expect others to take too much responsibility for their own emotions/actions," Mark Manson writes.

Here's the painful truth: My son's mother should have never let me marry her. The thought makes me squirm, knowing that my son wouldn't be here if that had been the case. But in the context of healthy relationships, letting that young woman cry while huddled on the floor should have been a one- or two-strike policy.

She needed to be loved in that moment. All I had to do was sit on the floor next to her. Maybe shut up and listen. Those were moments when she was down in a hole, and not only did I not jump in, too, but I didn't even give her the courtesy of jotting down a prayer to drop in there with her.

She was hurt and afraid, and I abandoned her because my priority was NOT being told what to do. Not letting someone else have power over me. Not being beholden to the emotional experiences of another person.

Love and intimacy and vulnerability and trust are about being able to surrender. And I wasn't ready to do that. And that young woman who deserved better should have told me to go fuck myself and left.

If my wife made a mistake, it was believing that I might organically grow out of whatever I was holding on to. From her perspective, I was either hurting her on purpose or hurting her in my blind spots. In either event, she shouldn't have let me get close enough to do either.

When people hurt us, we bear responsibility for getting ourselves out of harm's way. And just maybe, if she had done that, I would have begun my pursuit of empathy and emotional intelligence and the development of relationship skills much sooner in life. I'm not saying our divorce was my wife's fault. Of course, it wasn't. I'm saying the healthiest, wisest decision she could have made was not allowing someone who lacked empathy and emotional intelligence to marry her in the first place. She deserved better. I just didn't know it yet. And maybe she didn't either.

# CONCLUSION: THE ART
# OF GETTING TO TOMORROW

I WOKE UP IN AN EMPTY CONCRETE STAIRWELL. I DIDN'T KNOW
where I was. I was fully clothed but missing my shoes. I was frustrated as
I came to because I'd been trying to open a locked door, which I realized
later was the access door to the roof of the hotel I was staying in.

I was drugged and robbed during a work trip in Las Vegas, Nevada.
They took my phone, the cash I'd won playing blackjack, and the shoes
I'd been wearing. I learned later that they had cleaned out my checking
account through a series of ATM withdrawals and Venmo transfers, so
that was nice of me to share my banking PIN information with them.

Physically, I was fine. Which, in hindsight, seems fortunate. And
the truth is that I didn't have enough money for it to really have mattered other than a few weeks of inconvenience. *Hahaha! Joke's on you,
assholes!*

Mentally and emotionally, I was not fine. Something about the incident had triggered something in me and caught me by surprise. It felt
exactly like those initial weeks after divorce. *Everything is wrong.*

I couldn't describe it. None of my feelings made sense to me. Intellectually, I thought my body was overreacting. But our insides—all the

invisible stuff that makes us, us—have a funny way of not always doing what our brains think they should.

One minute I was with friends listening to a cheesy Vegas cover band in an open-air bar in the middle of The Golden Nugget. Then I left for a couple of minutes to use the restroom—and the very next thing I remember is waking up five hours later in a hotel stairwell several miles away, having apparently provided strangers with the private banking information and phone passcodes they needed to clean me out financially.

From a certain perspective, you could say I'm lucky to be alive, and that I'm fortunate to have ended up at my hotel, even if it were in a dingy metal and concrete emergency stairwell.

*But why do I feel this thing I don't have a name for?*

On the surface, it's a ridiculous comparison, right? Divorce is hugely disruptive. Your person leaves you. Your entire life changes overnight, forever. And this was not that.

*So why? Why is it feeling the same?*

Divorce was my first encounter with inner brokenness. It was my first true encounter with darkness. Things were heavy and ugly and painful and scary and broken, and there was nowhere to run.

That was its defining characteristic. That you took it with you everywhere, no matter what. It greeted you in the morning. It sat on your chest as you tried to fall back asleep in the middle of the night. It rode in the passenger seat next to you while you were driving around. It poked you and asked you to pay attention to it while you were trying to watch movies or sports. It inserted itself in your conversations with friends and family while you were just trying to have a good time like you had always done before.

It built and built and built until the only thing left to do was cry like a child.

And you kept waiting for it to go away, but every time you looked in the mirror, you could still see it hiding behind the dead eyes of the stranger in your reflection.

I don't know what to call this feeling or how to categorize it, so I've always just called it being broken. I was once a certain way—a way that felt normal and right. And then suddenly I was something else. I was a different way, and everything about it sucked more than the old way that I'd gotten used to for thirty-four years.

Finding my way back from that is one of the most difficult things I've done. It's perhaps my greatest personal achievement, because I didn't know the human body could feel like that and I didn't know whether coming back from it were possible.

But you do come back. And following that drugging and robbery, it was happening again. I was shaken, not just by the incident but by the idea that I was once again feeling things in the invisible places with no means of fixing them and nowhere to run away from them.

When everything is very bad, we're simply in survival mode, trying to return to a sense of normalcy.

I reminded myself, just as I would a coaching client or friend, that there is no Skip or Fast-Forward button to push. I reminded myself that the only way to get anywhere sustainable is the long way. The hard way.

As the superb writer and podcaster Glennon Doyle says, "*We can do hard things.*"

I remembered that I had only one job. Just one.

*Breathe.*

My only job was to breathe just one more breath. And once I'd completed that task, my only mission was to do that again.

*One more breath.*

When you breathe enough times today, tomorrow always comes.

And after enough tomorrows come, you find yourself further down the trail—finally a safe distance from the shitty, life-wrecking event you were trying to escape. Or maybe more accurately, you carried the shitty, life-wrecking event with you as you continued down the trail but you finally made peace with the idea of setting it down and moving forward without it.

I don't pretend to know.

I just think there's something important about breathing when it's difficult to do anything else.

**To recover from bad things, the three steps are:**

1. *Breathe.*
2. *Love yourself.*
3. *Repeat.*

I repeated it like a mantra after my wife left and I didn't know whether I'd wake up the next day or whether I even wanted to. Because if there were no hope of that feeling going away, the future wasn't looking very bright.

*Just breathe. Everything's going to be okay.*

It never happened as fast as I wanted it to because there are no hacks. No cheat codes. No magical work-arounds. There's just the long way through. Never easy, but always simple.

Breathe. Just one more time. I've breathed millions of times in my life with zero awareness that I was doing it. So, if I breathe purposefully? If I try hard? I'm confident I can always take one more.

And after breathing enough times, you get to be you again. You get to wake up tomorrow, where the best thing that ever happens to you might happen.

Tomorrow is a gift waiting to be opened. When you're ready.

*Breathe.*

You will be.

O

Maybe it goes away entirely one day. The toll from divorce. Maybe I'll eventually wake up and not feel it anymore.

At the time of this writing, it has been eight years. That seems like a lot. One more year, and we will have been divorced for as long as we were married.

I don't sit around pining for the life I had. I'm as "over it" as I'm going to get. I can go days, even weeks, without thinking about it. Days and weeks without feeling anything sad or painful. But sometimes I do.

Sometimes, I still have to hold back tears like a fake tough guy when my son is waving to me from the front window of his mom's house as I'm driving away.

Sometimes, I hear about our old friends whom I never see or talk to getting together with or going on vacation with my ex and her boyfriend. My brain says it's fine. I don't have any hard feelings about any of them. Even the boyfriend, who's a really solid guy whom I can trust to be good to her and to my son, which are invaluable things to be able to feel in a shared-parenting situation. But you still feel something less than fine.

And sometimes, I have a moment I could have never seen coming. There was a life and a story and a normalcy and a dream—an expectation, really—of the future, and there's so much safety and security and stability in having those things.

And divorce takes it away. The end—whether abrupt or from slow decay—takes away that life and that story and that normalcy and that dream. It drugs you and robs you of your safety and security. It leaves you confused and wanting to cry in a dingy, barren concrete stairwell trying to open a locked door that won't budge.

○

The most important work—the most important thing—I've ever done is to learn how to be grateful for that moment when I watched my wife and son drive away for the last time as I was sobbing and puking in my kitchen sink. Shaking. Cursing anyone and anything. Cursing everything.

Wanting to be dead because I didn't know you could be alive and feel THAT at the same time.

Angry with her. Angry with God. Angry with my parents. Angry with everyone who hid from me the truth about what it really takes to show up for someone else in a marriage.

Angry that I didn't love her enough. Angry that I didn't love myself enough.

And you stand alone in the quiet, empty house. Where there used to be sound and human connection and life, there was none.

No one tells you how loud the silence can be when you confront it for the first time. Where there's no one to distract you from the truth. Where there's nowhere to hide from yourself.

Every cell in your body screams to run and hide. That's all I wanted to do—move far away or to somewhere from my past where I'd be surrounded by family and friends. But there was a little boy, and that boy was my life. And for better or worse, by proxy, so was his mother. Everything had changed, but also, nothing had. There was no easy way out this time. Life was going to make me stare at what I'd done long enough for me to own it.

And so, you cry, because there's nothing left to do. You cry until there are no tears left. You vomit until you're dry heaving because there's nothing left to purge.

And then you get off the floor and try to live again.

*Just breathe.*

You breathe enough breaths to get to tomorrow. And then you choose to be courageous enough to do it again the next day. And then the one after that.

Only now you know how loud the silence can be. Now you know how good you had it. Now you know how severe invisible pain can hurt. Now you know what it feels like to not want to be alive anymore.

"When that happens to you," said David Foster Wallace to David Lipsky when discussing his experience of being in a mental institution on suicide watch, "you get tremendously, just unprecedentedly willing to examine other alternatives for how to live."

That was the gift my wife had given me. I became unprecedentedly willing to examine other ways for how to live.

○

I used to be a guy so certain of my decency and good intentions that I wouldn't consider the possibility that my words and actions could hurt someone else. Especially someone I loved.

But then I died—sobbing and dry heaving into the same sink next to which I would set the drinking glass that my wife and I used to argue about. In a very meaningful way, I died. And now I'm someone else.

And I mourn the loss of the person I used to be. That guy was happy all the time. That guy had a rich and vibrant social life. That guy was a fun guy to know, and a fun guy to be.

But he was also a threat. The person I used to be was a perpetual threat to hurt—to literally hurt—the people I loved and to believe that they were in the wrong if they dared to suggest that I had harmed them somehow.

The person I used to be didn't have a prayer of ever achieving a sustainable, healthy romantic relationship. The person I used to be was never going to be the kind of father my son could trust when life feels hard.

This is how your marriage ends. But, if you're willing to breathe enough times, if you're willing to examine alternatives for how to live, it's also how your life begins.

Divorce is the worst thing that ever happened to me. There is no close, second-place thing.

But now I get to be me. It's not easier. It's just better.

# ACKNOWLEDGMENTS

TO MY SON, THANK YOU FOR BEING AN AMAZING KID WHO EN-courages me to try to help others. I am so proud of you.

To my son's mother, thank you for supporting this process, treating me kindly, and being an extraordinary parenting partner despite any anxiety and resentment you may feel about it. You're an amazing mom and I'm grateful for you every day.

To my parents, stepparents, and siblings. Thank you for your love, support, and many sacrifices through the years. I only get to be me because of you.

To Mark Groves. Dude. I finally listened to you. And now we have a book! *What?!* You're smart. Thank you for the encouragement I needed to take the leap.

To Jancee Dunn. Thank you for reaching out to me and writing about my work. This book wouldn't exist without you.

To my editors Gideon Weil, Sam Tatum, and Maya Alpert, and the extraordinary bookmaking crew at HarperOne. Thank you so much for this opportunity and for helping me to make this book the best version of itself.

To my team of agents at Creative Artists Agency, but especially literary agents Anthony Mattero and Mollie Glick. You're the absolute best.

To former CAA agent and current entertainment executive Vanessa Silverton-Peel. You changed my life and I'll never forget it.

To my coaching clients who generously allowed me to share their personal stories throughout this book. I am so grateful for the opportunity to know you and work with you.

To the authors who inspire me and my work every day, especially Mark Manson, Eve Rodsky, Glennon Doyle, James Clear, Brené Brown, David Foster Wallace, and James Altucher. All of you are my heroes.

To my dear friend and attorney, BZ. Thank you for being there. Couldn't do this without you.

To my friends JH, AR, MDB, KS, SG, JL, AK, LW, JT, and CL. Thank you for reading and providing important feedback. Thank you for your support and encouragement as I was writing this, and always.

To longtime readers and social media followers of the blog *Must Be This Tall To Ride*. We did a thing! And I only believed it was possible because of you. Thank you for saving my life.